THE DYING PATIENT
A Supportive Approach

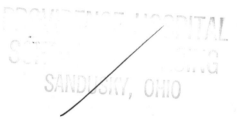

THE DYING PATIENT

A Supportive Approach

Edited by
Rita E. Caughill
R.N., M.S.

Associate Professor, Adult Health Nursing,
School of Nursing, State University of
New York at Buffalo

Little, Brown and Company
Boston

To my husband and children,
a legacy of love

CONTRIBUTING AUTHORS

Ruth A. Assell, R.N., M.S.
Assistant Professor, Community Health Nursing
College of Nursing, University of Kentucky, Lexington

Rita E. Caughill, R.N., M.S.
Associate Professor, Adult Health Nursing
School of Nursing, State University of New York at Buffalo

Ruth Gale Elder, R.N., Ph.D.
Associate Professor, School of Nursing and Sociology Department
State University of New York at Buffalo

Claudine R. Gartner, R.N., M.S.Ed.
Associate Professor, Maternal Child Health
College of Nursing, University of Kentucky, Lexington

Carol S. Green-Epner, R.N., M.S.
Assistant Professor, Child Health Nursing
School of Nursing, State University of New York at Buffalo

Clark Hopkins, Ph.D.
Professor Emeritus, Classical Art and Archeology
The University of Michigan, Ann Arbor

Carol Ren Kneisl, R.N., M.S.
Associate Professor
Graduate Program in Community Psychiatric Nursing
State University of New York at Buffalo

PREFACE

In recent years, health professionals at all levels have shown increasing concern about their roles in effectively meeting the needs of dying patients. With the ever-widening interval between initial diagnosis of a fatal illness and the final event of death, it becomes ever more important for caregivers to improve their relationships with the terminally ill.

All too often, medical and nursing personnel, intent upon the skills of physical care, ignore the basic psychological needs of the dying. This may be due partly to the fact that they do not really know what the patient's needs are, nor how to go about assessing those needs. An even larger factor, however, is the extreme discomfort experienced by most people in the presence of dying and of death. Nurses may suffer the same distress as everyone else since, unfortunately, few nurses are any better prepared than the lay person to cope with the realities of dying.

Despite the current proliferation of books dealing with various aspects of death, grief, and bereavement, there is little available for practicing nurses or nursing students, who are at the bedside of dying patients every day, to guide them in recognizing their responsibilities in the care of the dying. It is for such nurses that this book was written. It makes no claim to be a comprehensive text but is, rather, a supplementary book of readings. It is intended as a reference source to assist nursing personnel in developing the knowledge and skills they need in order to give thoughtful, supportive care to dying patients.

Throughout the book, the generic pronoun "she" is used frequently when referring to the nurse and "he" when referring to the patient or the physician. Obviously, nurses, patients, physicians, and all others are well represented by both sexes, but to state this fact repeatedly or to spell out both genders in every case becomes awkward and cumbersome.

To the many nursing students who originally inspired this volume by their insistence on more and more help in coping with the dying, I am exceedingly grateful. Special thanks are also due to those students whose clinical experiences formed the basis for some of the cases presented in the book.

For their critical review of portions of the manuscript, I am indebted to my colleagues, Miss Madeline Kennedy, Dr. Shirley Steele, and Mrs. Vera Harmon. Their comments and suggestions were always constructive and helpful. Additional editorial assistance was provided by Jim and Shelley Caughill and is most gratefully acknowledged.

Special thanks and gratitude are due Mrs. Patricia Brock, whose expert typing and skillful handling of the manuscript were essential to its completion. Her patience and dedication under the pressures of the final few weeks deserve particular praise and commendation.

My deepest gratitude to my family, who sacrificed innumerable hours of companionship, recreation, and togetherness, yet remained understanding and uncomplaining through the many long months the book was in preparation.

R. E. C.
Buffalo

CONTENTS

THE DYING PATIENT
PATIENT
A Supportive
Approach

Between Life and Death
There must somewhere be a harmony;
Otherwise the world
Could not have borne through the ages,
Smiling, such a cruel deceit,
And all the lights of her stars
Would have darkened!

Rabindranath Tagore, *A Flight of Swans*

1. DYING AND SOCIETY

Ruth Gale Elder

Death is a social and biological fact of life which affects not only the individual but the social arrangements and relationships in the human group to which he belongs. Every society has developed ways of managing death – of providing support for the bereaved, dispersing the property, recruiting new role replacements, and disposing of the body. Before modern times societies were highly oriented to this recurrent interruption, for death was an everyday event, frequently striking people with key roles in the community and thus disrupting the social order to a much greater extent than is the case today. As premature death becomes a problem of the past, new concerns arise to trouble us, issues connected with the management of the dying process itself. These issues involve the prolongation of life through our new technology, the right of man to accelerate his dying process, the right to freedom from pain at the cost of shortened days, the isolation and loneliness of those dying in our institutions, and the impersonal treatment of relatives as they struggle to cope with the last days of their beloved.

Society's Attitudes Toward Death
Changes in Life Expectancy
Before we can fully consider these topics, it may help to put them into historical perspective. One of the dramatic changes our society now faces is the prospect of the majority of people living into old age. The full meaning of the

Revised from Dying in the U.S.A., *International Journal of Nursing Studies* 10:171, 1973. With permission of Pergamon Press Ltd.

extension of average life expectancy is difficult to comprehend. It is changing our population structure, and it presents us with a complex of problems associated with old age, death, and dying that no society has ever faced before.

Fantastic as it may seem from our current vantage point, prehistoric man is believed to have lived only about eighteen years on the average, and is thought to have rarely survived beyond the age of forty [6]. Lerner [26] estimates that life expectancy in ancient Greece was probably about twenty years, and in ancient Rome, twenty-two years. By the time of the Middle Ages in England it had crept up to thirty-three years, and it was estimated to be in the vicinity of thirty-six years in the mid-seventeenth century. It was still only about forty years in England and America at the beginning of the last century, although by 1900 it had escalated to forty-seven years.

The truly dramatic changes in life expectancy took place relatively recently. As a consequence of the control of communicable diseases in the United States and the improvement of standards of living, life expectancy surged up to 54.5 years by 1915. It dipped violently in 1918 because of the great flu epidemic, but soon afterward it regained its steady climb. At the end of the 1930s it was 63.3 years, and by the end of the 1940s, in response to the discovery of antibiotics, it had spurted up to sixty-eight years. Subsequently the rapid increase tapered off. In the ensuing twenty years, life expectancy increased by only three years; the 1971 estimate was seventy-one years, ranging from 75.6 years for white females to 61.2 years for nonwhite males [30].

From this brief account it can be seen that life expectancy has been increasing since the beginning of recorded history and has accelerated with time. During the past 100 years, in the industrialized West, it has changed from approximately forty-five to approximately seventy years. Whereas half the population used to die before forty-five, half now lives beyond the age of seventy. As a consequence, the shape of the population profile has changed. In 1850 only 13 percent of the population was forty-five or older, but by 1950 one third of the population was in this age-group [38]. Inevitably the causes of death have changed, too. Earlier, death was primarily due to acute communicable diseases and gastrointestinal upsets. Now the primary causes of death are associated with old age, heart disease, cancer, and stroke.

Changes in Family Structure and Function
in Care of the Dying and Dead
In addition to the dramatic changes in the average age of death, the population pattern, and the causes of death, there are a number of other important social changes to consider if we are to understand what is happening today. The industrial revolution of the eighteenth and nineteenth centuries oriented the entire economy around the market and factory system instead of around the farm and the homestead. This fostered major changes in family structure and functions. Occupations were separated from family roles, and many functions such as education of the young, production of food and clothing, and care of the sick were shifted from the household into specialized institutions.

In colonial America most people were nursed at home and died there [4]. Death took place in the midst of kin, with the comfort of familiar surroundings and loved faces. The deathwatch was a family watch. After death it was generally the family's responsibility to care for the body, which was bathed and dressed for the last symbolic good-byes of friends and relatives. The body was kept at home until the funeral, and those who wished to pay their respects came to the family house to do so. Usually a relative sat up all night with the deceased. It was also the family, with the help of clergy and friends, who made all the funeral arrangements.

Today it is estimated that about three quarters of the deaths in the United States occur in institutions despite the fact that most people say they would rather die at home [26]. The general hospital is the most common location for death, although some deaths occur in nursing homes and mental hospitals. Those that do not take place in institutions are likely to be sudden, ranging from traumatic accidents to peaceful death in sleep. This means that the dying phase of life usually occurs in surroundings unfamiliar to the persons concerned. Dying is now likely to be managed by strangers, institutional personnel, rather than the family, and in some cases the family is not present at all.

After death the body is transferred from the hospital to the mortuary establishment, euphemistically called a funeral "home." There it is prepared for disposal by people hired especially for this purpose. The director of the mortuary establishment usually manages all the funeral arrangements for the family and with his questions and suggestions strongly influences the types of procedures to be performed, the casket to be ordered, and the clothing to be purchased.* The family home usually is bypassed entirely, for the body is then placed in a special room called the "funeral parlor." All the visiting by family and friends takes place in this relatively impersonal atmosphere, and the behavior of the mourners is restricted to that permitted by the policies of the funeral home.

Funerals, too, have changed. They used to be important events in the life of the community, serving the functions of rites of passage, celebrating the transition to a new state of being and at the same time heightening group cohesion by reaffirming the importance of the remaining group to its members, as well as providing a means of disposing of the body [9]. Nowadays funerals are less extensive. The average person attends few of them apart from those of his immediate family, until he is elderly himself. Formal observances are completed in a shorter time, possibly because there is less demand for magical precautions and religious rituals in an increasingly secular society, which has decreasing belief in ghosts and religious afterlife. Also a shortened service is often considered essential by those engaged in the competitive work demands of a complex urban society, focused on conserving time whenever possible.

Consequences of the Changes
The separation of dying and death from the family has a number of consequences. It relieves the family of respon-

---

*Embalming is so taken for granted in the United States that few people apart from those of certain religious faiths realize that it is optional, and the funeral director does not usually present it in such a way as to imply a choice.

sibilities many persons have found onerous, even odious. It also minimizes the extent to which death interrupts the orderly structuring of everyday life. It can also have negative consequences due to the impersonality of the people and settings associated with its management.

The modern hospital, as an organization, is committed to the routinization of the handling of life and death crises [2]. As a consequence many people are needlessly isolated and lonely when they become patients in hospitals during their last days. Sudnow [47], for example, reported that most patients in the county hospital he studied died unattended. In part this was due to the tactics of personnel, who were attempting to minimize the disruption death made in their other ward responsibilities. They encouraged family members to go home and wait for news of death or at least to wait outside in the corridors and not in the patient's room. Separation of the family from the patient made management of the last phase of life easier, because traditional nursing practices, the comfort and care procedures, were regarded as less important at this time and could be omitted more readily if family members were not present.

Encountering depersonalized approaches in connection with the sacred aspects of life is likely to promote feelings of frustration, despair, bitterness, and alienation. Duff and Hollingshead [7] describe the anguish experienced by a woman ushered out of her dying husband's room shortly before his death. "Why couldn't I have seen him before he died?" she cried, when she was later approached to give permission for an autopsy. The bureaucratization of death has high psychological costs unless personnel remain sensitive to the meaning of events for both patients and families.

American Attitudes Toward Death

The literature on attitudes toward death in American society is both contradictory and critical. At one extreme Americans are criticized for their propensity to deny death [17], and at the other they are criticized for focusing on it too much [29]. Funerals are seen as either costly, vulgar, and unnecessary or as necessary but insufficient. Depending on which set of literature one chooses, one can gain an image of a people obsessed with death or oblivious to it [31].

Numerous authors describe the culture as *death-denying.* Elaborate psychological theories have been developed to explain death denial [3, 51], but the evidence to support these theories is primarily based on illustrations which are either idiosyncratic or more readily explained in another way. Denial to one man is religion to another. Fulton [12] speaks of euphemisms of denial such as "passing away," "gone home," and "gone beyond," but one can question whether use of these phrases necessarily indicates denial of death. Death as a transition or journey is a very old belief, and as it is difficult to bring specific evidence to bear as to whether another existence does lie beyond death, one could just as easily argue that those who suggest that death is the absolute end are denying the reality of a passage to an afterlife. Furthermore, as Dumont and Foss [8] have recently noted, one can also point to expressions which do not soften the reality of death, such as "kicked the bucket," "croaked," and "bit the dust."

Cosmetic preparation of the corpse in America is often cited as evidence of the death-denying propensities of this culture. This same custom, however, can also be used as evidence for the acceptance of death, for the body is arranged so that it is the center of attention — death is highlighted. A number of alternative explanations for such customs may be more valid than the death-denial hypothesis. For example, there may be a desire on the part of family and friends to give viewers a good last impression of the deceased, which would remind them of how he was prior to the ravages of the last illness. Viewing the body in this way is not necessarily conducive to denial of death but instead to facing death. Pine [34] argues that our expensive funeral practices are a means of expressing sentiments rather than denying death. He considers them to be a substitute for many of the social arrangements and ceremonies of the past, which allowed people to express their feelings about the deceased publicly and directly. Then, too, we should not forget that the funeral industry works hard to sell the elaborate preparation of the body, and some people may simply succumb to salesmanship strategies. Just because a behavior pattern exists does not necessarily mean that those who participate in it endorse it wholeheartedly or want it to continue.

Information about the attitudes of the elderly has been available for some time. Contrary to the hypothesized tendency to deny death, most studies indicate that old people think about death, are willing to talk about it, and have made preparations for it. Few show marked fear of it, and the prevailing view is one of acceptance. Those in poor health tend actually to look forward to it [49]. Riley [37], in a survey of a cross section of the United States adult population, found that these views were not confined to the elderly but were held by a majority of the people in the sample studied. Most of these respondents also thought that death was not as tragic for the one who dies as for those left behind. Only a small proportion thought of death in terms of suffering, and most subscribed to the idea that it is sometimes a blessing. Assuming the pervasiveness of a death taboo, Riley hypothesized that many people would be reluctant to make arrangements for death, but this was not supported by the data. Over 80 percent of the respondents thought it preferable to make some sort of plan for death, and approximately one half said that they had made a point of talking about death with those closest to them.

Given the current mortality and life-expectancy statistics, a lack of concern about death is reasonable. Current data seem to support Parsons's contention [33] that the major orientation in America is to accept death as normal at the end of the life cycle. Death is upsetting primarily when it occurs prematurely or is accompanied by suffering or violence, for premature death and suffering are no longer accepted as natural in this society. In addition death is no longer of great concern in our society because it does not seriously affect the work that has to be done. Most deaths take place after the productive years of life are over. Even when death comes earlier, there is little disruption, because work is now organized in such a way that our major institutions are relatively independent of the individuals who carry out the roles within them [2].

The affective ties within the small nuclear family are the most vulnerable to disruption through death, because intensity of feeling is distributed to a relatively small number of people, and it is difficult to replace these emotional bonds quickly. Because most deaths take place among the elderly, however, and the elderly are relatively segregated — that is, they are not usually members of the nuclear family — the burden of emotional suffering most frequently falls on the elderly themselves, when they lose their partners and friends. Thus, the hypothesis that this is a death-denying culture lacks substantial empirical support, and absence of concern about death can be more easily explained in other ways. Indeed, Parsons [33] considers those groups that tend to deny certain aspects of the reality of death (fundamentalist and positive-thinking groups) to have deviant orientations which are not representative of the mainstream of American life. Further study is needed to ascertain more clearly the existing variations in orientation and the relative prevalence of those that could be described legitimately as death-denying. This is a vast country stratified in many different ways, and further research may reveal that conflicting beliefs on this subject arise from differences in attitudes peculiar to specific subgroups.

Death in the Hospital
What People Want Regarding Their Own Deaths
Fulton [12, 13] indicates that people prefer to die quickly, painlessly, and with as little fuss and inconvenience to their loved ones as possible. They prefer to be at home when they die, and they want to be surrounded by family and

friends. Feifel [11], in one of his most recent studies, reported that the terminally ill had a more urgent desire for the emotional bulwark of family and home than did the seriously ill, but that both these groups emphasized the importance of the family more than did a control group of healthy normals. Feifel's work has been supported by a number of other studies which indicate the importance of the family to people under stress [50]. The closer people feel to personal death, the more important become those people and places representing love and psychological security.

There have been comparatively few studies of dying patients, partly because it has been thought that discussion of death would upset them. Feifel, who was one of the first to conduct major research on the thoughts and feelings of dying patients, reported extreme opposition from administrators and physicians [10]. When he attempted to gain access to the patients in order to conduct interviews, he was asked, "Isn't it cruel, sadistic, and traumatic to discuss death with seriously and terminally ill people?" He soon discovered, however, that patients were glad to talk to him, and that they found the interviews supportive rather than destructive. They even thanked him for the opportunity to examine their feelings about death. Despite this, frustrating blocks continued to be placed in Feifel's way as he attempted to conduct his research, and this led him to believe that death was a taboo topic, at least among health professionals. Kübler-Ross also has reported strong objections to her beginning efforts to talk with dying patients [25].

Feifel found that both the sick and the healthy said that they would definitely want to be informed if they had an incurable disease. "It's my life, I have a right to know," was the usual attitude, in combination with the themes of being able to prepare for the end and being able to spend the remaining time in some preferred way. This result was similar to that found in a number of studies which indicate that the overwhelming majority of patients want to know the truth about their diagnosis or, if they have been already told of a fatal diagnosis, approve of having been told [1, 14, 21, 42].

Physicians are much less likely to want to inform patients of an unfavorable prognosis than patients would wish. Oken [32] found that 88 percent of the 219 physicians whom he studied preferred not to tell cancer patients of an unfavorable prognosis. Furthermore a significant proportion of these physicians indicated that their approach was not likely to be changed by the results of research, which suggests that the basis on which many of these decisions are made is emotional rather than rational. Physicians may have relaxed to some extent about deliberately keeping the truth from patients, but Feifel's work indicates [11] that they are still much more reluctant to inform patients than patients are about being informed. Kram and Caldwell [24] also found that general physicians, more than any of the other four professional groups they studied (lawyers, psychiatrists, Protestant ministers, rabbis), recommended evasion rather than telling the patient the truth.

There is strong evidence that those working with dying patients find talking about death very trying and avoid it if at all possible [18, 20]. Quint [35] vividly described the pain and emotional upset professionals experience when they permit patients with cancer to talk openly about their concerns. The medical field's strong emphasis on preserving life may make health professionals unfit for dealing with the dying patient, if it means that death makes them feel like failures. Kastenbaum [19] thinks that physicians *need* to deny the possibility of their patients' death, because otherwise they would lose interest in caring for them. Crane [5] speculates that the physician's motive in curtailing information may be to maintain control over the doctor-patient relationship, as the patient who is aware of his fate may be more difficult to handle. However, it may simply be that through avoiding talk about death, physicians hope to avoid inflicting unnecessary pain and genuinely believe that they are acting in the patient's best interest. They also may not feel equipped to deal with the emotional scenes that sometimes follow informing the patient. It is not an easy task to support a patient through the phases of anger, depression, and grief which often follow the disclosure that death is imminent, and most physicians, and nurses, too, have had little training for it.

This raises the question of the patient's right to know the truth and whose right it is to decide whether he *should* know. Even if knowing were expected to have negative consequences, can this be considered a sufficient reason for preventing a patient who wants to know his diagnosis from knowing it? This question goes beyond the realm of the health professions. It is a societal question concerning the extent of an individual's right to have control over his body and knowledge about himself to the extent that it is available. Given the indications that physicians have both a greater reluctance than other professionals to inform patients honestly and a higher resistance to facing death than the average person [11], they may be the least qualified to make this type of decision.

Awareness Context

Whether or not the patient is aware of his diagnosis is of crucial importance to nursing personnel who bear the brunt of day-to-day interaction with patients. Glaser and Strauss [15, 46] have given detailed descriptions of the effect of "who knows about the possibilities of death" on staff-patient interaction and patient care. *Awareness context* was the term Glaser and Strauss used to represent this component of the environment, and they found that four contexts were particularly important in the dying situations they studied. The first, which they labeled *closed-awareness context,* was one in which the staff knew the patient's diagnosis but the patient did not, a situation with which most nurses are familiar.

The second was a *suspicion context,* in which the dying person suspected the truth, while the staff continued to act out the fiction that recovery was expected. The third was described as a *pretense context,* and meant that both patient and staff were fully aware of the impending death, realized that the other was also aware, and yet acted as if the patient would eventually get better. The fourth context, found rather infrequently, was one of *open awareness.* Both parties in this situation were aware of the impending death, and discussed it openly.

Glaser and Strauss noted that the *closed-awareness* context provoked a striking division of labor. The management of communication and actions designed to keep the patient in ignorance of his health status was left almost entirely to the nursing staff. Physicians focused on technical aspects of care and, by keeping their visits to a minimum, escaped the problems of conducting conversations in which death was to be avoided.

These researchers observed several characteristics of the death situation which made it possible for staff to maintain a closed-awareness context for comparatively long periods of time. The patients were usually unfamiliar with the signs of impending death and therefore accepted with little question the explanations the staff gave about disturbing symptoms or failure to regain strength. Also, the patients had no allies to help them find out the truth, for families and fellow patients hesitated to inform them if they thought the physician would disapprove. In addition to this the hospital staff was skilled at withholding information and had long training to act collusively around patients so as not to reveal medical secrets. Records were kept out of reach, and patients were reprimanded if they tried to read them. Professional rationales for withholding information (such as a belief that one should not deny hope) played a part by making the staff feel guilty if they revealed information that allowed the patient to suspect the truth.

Over and above all this the staff used a number of "situation as normal" interaction tactics. They acted as if the patient were not dying but only ill, and they talked about the future as if it were certain that the patient would have a part in it. They told stories about other patients who had

had similar conditions but were now well. They even assured patients directly that they would live, fabricating "for the patient's own good" [15, 36].

In order to manage all this staff members have to be extremely alert as to just how they are answering all the patient's remarks and questions. They have to manage facial expressions and gestures carefully so as not to give the show away. They have to control any sadness they feel about the patient's approaching death. Little wonder that under such exhausting conditions they almost invariably reduce the amount of time they spend with the patient, or restrict their conversations. If the situation goes on long enough, the closed context usually begins to break down. Patients start to pick up signals and cues which indicate that all is not well, and the context shifts into one of *suspicion, pretense,* or *open awareness.*

Glaser and Strauss point out that each type of context has many implications for both patient and staff. The closed-awareness context, for example, means that the patient cannot talk to his loved ones about his fate nor help them bear their grief. He is not in a position to consider what to do in his remaining time or prepare himself realistically for his demise. He cannot make decisions about bringing his life to a close or make plans which could affect others long after his death.

The closed context also has consequences for staff and family. They may be saved from stressful scenes that sometimes accompany the realization of impending death, but they also may lose the patient's trust as he becomes aware of deception. They are blocked from participating in what can be an enriching experience in life. Relatives cannot openly say goodbye to their loved ones or reminisce freely about the experiences they have shared together. They cannot as easily support nor share their feelings of grief with the dying person. They also cannot involve their loved ones in the plans which have to be made for the future, after death has taken place. Although some of these items may be irrelevant in particular situations, they can be important, even vital, in others.

The Dying Trajectory
The *dying trajectory* is a term used by Glaser and Strauss [16] to refer to the perceived course of death. One can speak of *quick* dying trajectories, *lingering* trajectories, and *uncertain* trajectories, each with its own set of hazards and opportunities. Expected quick deaths are probably the easiest for the staff to deal with. Unexpected quick deaths and lingering deaths are more difficult. In the current system of patient care lingering trajectories are probably the most difficult of all for both patients and staff.

Levine and Scotch [27] feel that the key to understanding the social consequences and problems of dying lies in time: the hours, days, months, and even years that it takes for the career of many terminal patients to unfold. Certainly as one scans the literature, one of the major areas in which problems seem to be heightened is in the care of the patient who is dying of cancer. What are the critical differences between dying of a condition such as cancer and dying of another kind of condition such as heart disease? At first glance it might seem to be the stigma associated with cancer, since people frequently react to cancer as being an "unclean" disease in contrast to, for example, heart disease. Or is it the fear of mutilation associated with cancer? On the other hand perhaps it is the long time factor, the *lingering trajectory* in Strauss's terms, which exhausts the resources of patients and staff, unless steps are deliberately taken to keep them replenished.

One of the major problems associated with cancer is the interruption of free and open communication between patient, family, and medical team. Despite the many studies of the 1950s [44, 48] indicating the extreme need of these patients for clearer communications and warm supportive relations from both staff and families, recent studies indicate that when such care is provided, it is still more the exception than the rule [7, 45, 47]. Duff and Hollingshead [7], in their study of a well-known teaching hospital, for example, found that the staff routinely attempted to maintain a closed-awareness context when dealing with cancer patients. They reported that evasions about diagnosis, prognosis, and the worth of treatment were the *rule* in serious illnesses rather than the exception, and that a patient with cancer had to make a determined effort to learn of the diagnosis. Probable prognosis was guarded even more closely than diagnosis, and the patients' questions were glossed over and evaded. The majority of the patients were highly suspicious if not actually aware of their diagnosis, but they did not share this with the staff or their families because of the evasions which characterized all communications. The primary effect of hospital staff efforts to maintain a closed-awareness context seems to be

breakdown in communications which promote in the
patient feelings of abandonment, rejection, depression, and
despair. Isolation may be one of the most painful psychological experiences associated with terminal illness.

Sometimes more than psychological estrangement is involved. Duff and Hollingshead reported that both patients
and families were confused by the physicians' and nurses'
evasions and fictions, and, as a consequence, much unnecessary physical suffering was endured. The patients agreed
to treatments and operations without realizing that they
were merely palliative and that there was little hope for
cure. Patients low in the socio-economic scale were the
least informed of all; not one was told that his illness was
terminal, and family members were told only when the
patients were near death [7].

Nonaccountability
Part of the problem in the care of the dying may lie in what
Glaser and Strauss call the *nonaccountability* of the psychosocial aspects of patient care. Personnel are accountable
institutionally and sometimes legally for certain aspects of
patient care such as diagnosis, treatment, carrying out the
technical procedures ordered, and physical care. Actions
taken in relation to them must be communicated to others
through either written or verbal reports. Neglect of any of
these aspects of care is therefore visible, subject to inquiry,
and possibly correctable. The socio-emotional components
of care, however, are not accountable in most hospital
situations. They are *not* generally inquired into, reported,
or discussed systematically. Even if personnel notice that

a patient is upset and report this to others, they seldom record the action taken in response to the patient's distress or the results they have obtained. Both successful and unsuccessful handling of traumatic situations are equally invisible, and neither are held in high esteem. Under these circumstances it is not surprising that accountable, and therefore highly visible, tasks have high priority, whereas nonaccountable, low-visibility tasks have low priority, if they are tended to at all. If a task becomes accountable, then an explanation is due if it is not carried out, and this in itself creates pressure for its completion [28].

Because the management of the socio-emotional components of patient care are nonaccountable, the quality of the interaction that takes place between patient and staff may depend more on such idiosyncratic matters as the personal and social characteristics of the people involved than on institutionalized methods of developing, maintaining, and improving this aspect of care. Although there is lip service given to the importance of the socio-emotional role, no means have been institutionalized of making it accountable and thus more visible. Matters probably will remain this way until clinical supervisors take systematic notice of how much the staff knows about the patient's reaction to his situation and his concern about his illness, care, and treatment and how well the staff responds to the patient's signals of distress. In-service education programs probably are required for both supervisors and staff before change in this area can be realistically expected, and changes in administrative priorities, policies, and practices as well as in clinical care undoubtedly will be involved.

A few studies indicate that vast changes in ward culture and staff performance can be accomplished through the assignment of consultants with specialized knowledge and training in working with the psychosocial components of care. Klagsburn [22], a psychiatrist, describes dramatic changes in the total ward culture, staff behavior, and patient behavior, as well as improvement in staff morale and capability, as a consequence of weekly discussions with the staff over an eighteen-month period. The discussion focused on problems of working with chronically ill patients with cancer and the staff's emerging ideas about how to improve the quality of life on the ward. This whole experiment was instigated by the head nurse who, realizing that the staff was unable to meet patient needs and that turnover was high on her unit, called for a consultant. Whether similar results can be obtained by professionals with less or different training, such as clinical specialists in nursing with master's or baccalaureate degrees, is an open question but an important one, as it is unrealistic to believe that there are sufficient psychiatrists to deal with the number of personnel in need of assistance with their programs in patient care.

Ambiguousness of Norms

Part of the dilemma in the care of the dying is the lack of explicit norms in our culture to guide the relationships between patients, family, and staff in the dying situation. Duff and Hollingshead [7] noted that each of these groups functioned within a framework of ambiguous assumptions as to "what must be done . . . what should be done . . . what could be done." The dramatic changes which have taken place in the last fifty years in the care of the dying, especially the shift in location from home to hospital, have been accomplished without concurrent development and institutionalization of customs and norms which guarantee humane, warm, supportive care.

Conversations with dying patients seem particularly difficult for health professionals. The common query of the neophyte is, "What should I say if he says he thinks he's dying?" Why is talking about death so difficult for these professionals; is it simply that they have not faced their own fears of dying and death? Is it connected with the death denial which some suggest is so predominant in our culture? Or is it that they lack guidelines, norms, and professional methods of proceeding which would enable them more adequately to converse with and thus understand the particular needs of the patient with whom they are dealing?

It should be remembered that talking about death falls within what Parsons calls the context of *privatization* [33]. It is one of those topics which is considered to be private, along with such other topics as personal finances, religious convictions, sexual habits, political activities, and strong emotions. Unless there is legitimate reason for inquiry, entering this area without invitation can be seen as a violation of the sacredness of the self. Consequently professional personnel usually bring with them from the common culture a hesitancy to intrude into such private areas as the patient's thoughts and feelings about emotion-ridden events.

In addition to this, recent generations are not as familiar with death because it so seldom occurs within the family home, for as noted earlier, it is mainly old people who die, and they are not as likely to be members of the nuclear household. Then, too, because of the relative infrequency of death among the young, there is little opportunity to learn how to deal with premature dying, which is almost always very upsetting in a society that places strong emphasis on the emotional importance of the relatively few members of the nuclear family, who are not easily replaced. Because young professionals are so inexperienced with this phase of life,* they usually require special preparation in order to come to terms with their own reactions to dying and death, particularly premature death. They need opportunities to gain facility in interacting with dying patients and to become clear about when it is appropriate, even essential, to set aside culturally acquired reticences in order to fulfill their professional role and potential as human beings.

Another item that is often overlooked is the importance of clarity about the purposes or goals of care. Sometimes the primary problem in care of the dying is that staff behavior is guided by norms associated with goals of curing or prolonging life, rather than those associated with goals of improving the quality of the last days. As Saunders [43] points out, when active treatment becomes irrelevant to the patient's real needs, then care of the patient should change to focus on comfort, making the patient's life as peaceful, contented, and meaningful as possible until he dies. At the

---

*In a recent study of health professionals Knutson [23] found that fewer than one third had been personally exposed to death. Only 15 percent had actually witnessed a death prior to professional training, and this was usually an accident.

point that comfort becomes the primary goal of care, the nursing professional can legitimately claim ascendancy in the management of care, for patient comfort has traditionally been one of the areas in which nursing has claimed special expertise. Unfortunately actions have not always lived up to the claims, for one still encounters withholding of pain medication for fear the patient may become addicted or death may be unduly hastened, even when addiction no longer matters and death is preferred to further pain. The nurse also gets caught up in resuscitation efforts long after the patient no longer wishes to be resuscitated. More study and strong stands are required if nursing is to move into a central position in the management of humane care for the dying, a position only too often occupied by no one at present. If both the medical profession and the nursing profession were willing, an *expanded* role for the nurse directed at maintaining the patient's comfort and capability as he desired it could be developed. It would require additional preparation in learning how to manage medications in the control of pain, as outlined by Saunders [43], and in learning how to assess and meet the needs of the dying patients and their families more adequately than is now the case.

A Broader Perspective

Death remains a tragic feature of life. It probably poses less of a problem for Western society today than it ever has in the past, because it does not, on the average, occur so early in life. But there appear to be more conflicts and dilemmas associated with dying than ever before. This is because increasing numbers die in institutions, apart from their families and friends.

We make a mistake, however, if we attribute the inadequacies of care of the dying solely to our feelings about dying and death. Studies of hospital situations in which death is *not* an issue reveal similar pictures of the staff's incomprehension of the patient's experience. Communication difficulties and insensitivity to patients' needs have been reported in outpatient departments [40], rehabilitation units [41], psychiatric units [39], and medical units [7]. For example, Duff and Hollingshead [7] reported that only a small proportion of the nurse respondents in their study knew anything about their patients' thoughts and feelings concerning their illness. The nurse-patient relationship was described as being technical, administrative, and task oriented. It was not person oriented. Patients did not feel that they could talk to their physicians either. Yet these patients often felt desperately anxious in the hospital situation. Their major source of solace was other patients, for their anguish and fears were outside the interests of the professional personnel.

The problem of providing adequate care for the dying is part of a much broader issue — the depersonalization associated with many of our large bureaucratic organizations today. We are really considering the problems provoked by the rapid changes which have taken place in our complex, industrialized society and the impersonality associated with the institutions which have evolved. Our schools, our prisons, our hospitals, our old age homes, our psychiatric centers, all are problematic in that clients in these places

tend to be treated like nonpersons, like objects on an as-
sembly line. This problem is highlighted by dying patients,
because they seem so little able to protect themselves and
because we have so many feelings about death and dying
ourselves.

One of our tasks, then, is to help personalize and human-
ize these complex service organizations in our society. We
cannot tackle them all, but we can take on the responsibility
of studying and attempting to change the ones in which we
work — hospitals, nursing homes, nursing schools, and universities. How can we reorganize our work so that the
environment is beneficial rather than noxious, so that our
responses are helpful rather than alienating? Perhaps it is
too much to expect hospitals that are currently geared to
technologically life-saving activities to devote part of their
resources to improving the quality of living for the dying.
If this is so, then it behooves us to establish special facilities
geared specifically to developing a ward climate which
allows patients to live until they die in the way they wish
and provides their relatives with whatever support they
require to sustain them, as they cope with this aspect of
life.

References

1. Aitken-Swan, V., and Easson, E. Reactions of cancer patients on
   being told their diagnosis. *Br. Med. J.* 1:779, 1959.
2. Blauner, R. Death and social structure. *Psychiatry* 29:378, 1966.
3. Borkenau, F. The Concept of Death. In Fulton, R. (Ed.), *Death
   and Identity.* New York: Wiley, 1965. P. 42.
4. Bowman, L. *The American Funeral.* Washington, D.C.: Public
   Affairs Press, 1959.

5. Crane, D. Dying and Its Dilemmas as a Field of Research. In Brim, O., et al. (Eds.), *The Dying Patient*. New York: Russell Sage, 1970.

6. Dublin, L. I. *The Facts of Life – From Birth to Death*. New York: Macmillan, 1951.

7. Duff, R. A., and Hollingshead, A. *Sickness and Society*. New York: Harper & Row, 1968.

8. Dumont, R. G., and Foss, C. F. *The American View of Death*. Cambridge, Mass.: Schenkman, 1972.

9. Durkheim, E. *The Elementary Forms of Religious Life*. New York: Macmillan, 1926, pp. 389–403.

10. Feifel, H. Death. In Farberow, N. L. (Ed.), *Taboo Topics*. New York: Atherton, 1963.

11. Feifel, H. Perception of death. *Ann. N.Y. Acad. Sci.* 164:19, 1969.

12. Fulton, R. The Sacred and the Secular: Attitudes of the American Public toward Death, Funerals, and Funeral Directors. In Fulton, R. (Ed.), *Death and Identity*. New York: Wiley, 1965. Pp. 89–105.

13. Fulton, R., and Gilbert, G. Death and Social Values. In Fulton, R. (Ed.), *Death and Identity*. New York: Wiley, 1965. Pp. 65–75.

14. Gerle, B., et al. The patient with inoperable cancer from the psychiatric and social standpoints: A study of 101 cases. *Cancer* 13:1206, 1960.

15. Glaser, B. G., and Strauss, A. L. *Awareness of Dying*. Chicago: Aldine, 1965.

16. Glaser, B. G., and Strauss, A. L. *Time for Dying*. Chicago: Aldine, 1968.

17. Gorer, G. *Death, Grief and Mourning: A Study of Contemporary Society*. New York: Doubleday, 1965.

18. Kalish, R. A. Aged and the dying process: The inevitable decision. *J. Soc. Issues* 21:88, 1965.

19. Kastenbaum, R. The realm of death: An emerging area of psychological research. *J. Human Relations* 13:538, 1965.

20. Kastenbaum, R., and Aisenberg, R. *The Psychology of Death.* New York: Springer, 1972.
21. Kelly, W. D., and Friesen, S. R. Do cancer patients want to be told? *Surgery* 27:822, 1950.
22. Klagsburn, S. Cancer, nurses, and emotions. *R.N.* 33:46, 1970.
23. Knutson, A. Cultural Beliefs in Life and Death. In Brim, O., et al. (Eds.), *The Dying Patient.* New York: Russell Sage, 1970.
24. Kram, C., and Caldwell, J. The dying patient. *Psychosomatics* 10:293, 1969.
25. Kübler-Ross, E. *On Death and Dying.* New York: Macmillan, 1969.
26. Lerner, M. When, Why and Where People Die. In Brim, O., et al. (Eds.), *The Dying Patient.* New York: Russell Sage, 1970.
27. Levine, S., and Scotch, N. Dying as an Emerging Social Problem. In Brim, O., et al. (Eds.), *The Dying Patient.* New York: Russell Sage, 1970. Pp. 211–224.
28. Merton, R. *Social Theory and Social Structure.* New York: Free Press of Glencoe, 1957. Pp. 374–379.
29. Mitford, J. *The American Way of Death.* New York: Simon & Schuster, 1963.
30. National Center for Health Statistics. *Vital Statistics of the United States, 1971.* Vol. II (Suppl. 5) Div. of Health, Education, and Welfare, Pub. No. 74-1147, 1974, p. 4.
31. Nettler, G. Review essay: On death and dying. *Soc. Probl.* 14:335, 1967.
32. Oken, D. What to tell cancer patients. *J.A.M.A.* 175:1120, 1968.
33. Parsons, T. Death in American society — A brief working paper. *Am. Behav. Scientist* 6:61, 1963.
34. Pine, V. Social organization of death. *Omega* 3:149, 1972.
35. Quint, J. Institutionalized practices of information control. *Psychiatry* 28:119, 1965.
36. Quint, J. The threat of death: Some consequences for patients and nurses. *Nurs. Forum* 8:286, 1969.

37. Riley, J. W. What People Think about Death. In Brim, O., et al. (Eds.), *The Dying Patient.* New York: Russell Sage, 1970.

38. Riley, J. W., and Foner, A. *Aging and Society.* New York: Russell Sage, 1969. Vol. I, pp. 22–23.

39. Rosenhan, D. L., et al. On being sane in insane places. *Science* 179:250, 1973.

40. Roth, J. Staff and client control strategies in urban hospital emergency services. *Urban Life and Culture* 1:39, 1972.

41. Roth, J., and Eddy, E. *Rehabilitation for the Unwanted.* New York: Atherton, 1967.

42. Samp, R. J., and Curreri, A. R. Questionnaire survey on public cancer education obtained from cancer patients and their families. *Cancer* 10:382, 1957.

43. Saunders, C. The last stages of life. *Am. J. Nurs.* 65:70, 1965.

44. Shands, H. C., et al. Psychological mechanisms in patients with cancer. *Cancer* 4:1159, 1951.

45. Simmons, S., and Given, B. Nursing care of the terminal patient. *Omega* 3:217, 1972.

46. Strauss, A., and Glaser, B. *Anguish.* Mill Valley, Calif.: Sociology Press, 1970.

47. Sudnow, D. *Passing On: The Social Organization of Dying.* Englewood Cliffs, N.J.: Prentice-Hall, 1967.

48. Sutherland, A., and Orbach, C. Psychological impact of cancer and cancer surgery: II. Depressive reactions associated with surgery. *Cancer* 6:958, 1953.

49. Swenson, W. Attitudes toward death among the aged. *Minn. Med.* 42:399, 1959.

50. Titmuss, R. M. *Problems of Social Policy.* London: Longmans, Green, 1950.

51. Wahl, C. The fear of death. *Bull. Menninger Clin.* 22:214, 1958.

2. GRIEVING: A RESPONSE TO LOSS

Carol Ren Kneisl

Bereavement, like death, is a universal and inevitable experience. We are most familiar with grief as an adaptational response to the loss, through death or separation, of a loved person. Grieving also occurs following the loss of anything, tangible or intangible, that is highly valued — a material possession, a position of status, a body part, a home, or a country, for example — and an understanding of the reactions common to loss in general will help in understanding grief reactions in response to the loss of a loved person through death. This chapter will not focus upon the dying person and his grief, as the other chapters do, but rather it will focus on those persons bereaved by death — by the loss of another.

Like most other universal and inevitable experiences, mourning has been treated historically as an accepted state of affairs, little thought about and even less understood, by professionals in the health sciences. Mental health professionals originally were interested in grieving when it became psychopathological or led to depression. Scattered throughout the psychological and psychiatric literature are a number of references to grieving from a psychoanalytical point of view in relation to depressive psychosis, agitated depression, or as a psychopathological response in time of war. Few were interested in exploring or seeking to understand the grieving process that is a necessary concomitant of activities of daily living. Some of the rare exceptions are to be found in the works of poets and philosophers — Homer, the Greek and Roman tragedians, Shakespeare, Milton, Dostoevski, Goethe, and more contemporarily Pinter, Albee, and O'Neill.

Cobb and Lindemann's [4] well-known therapeutic efforts following Boston's Cocoanut Grove nightclub fire with bereaved disaster victims and their families is the forerunner of more recent concerns for those who mourn. Shortly thereafter, Lindemann [8] expanded his observations to include the bereaved in various other more common settings. This classic work identified acute grief as a definite syndrome with psychological or somatic symptomatology, which may appear immediately or be delayed, exaggerated, or apparently absent. Distortions of the typical syndrome, which can be successfully transformed into a normal grief reaction with resolution, were also identified.

The Grieving Process
Normal Grieving Process
According to Lindemann there are five general classes of symptoms of normal grief. The first, somatic distress occurring in waves lasting from twenty minutes to one hour, is characterized by deep sighing respirations that are most conspicuous when the individual is discussing his grief, lack of strength, loss of appetite and sense of taste, tightness in the throat, and a choking sensation accompanied by shortness of breath. When the bereaved person learns that these uncomfortable experiences are precipitated by discussion of the circumstances surrounding bereavement and by receiving sympathy, he tends to try to avoid the syndrome at all costs. Avoidance is achieved through limiting interpersonal encounters, thereby increasing interpersonal distance from others, and by deliberately excluding from the thought process all references to the deceased.

The second general class of symptoms is preoccupation with the image of the deceased. This phenomenon is similar to daydreaming and is usually accompanied by a slight sense of unreality. Lindemann tells of a patient whose daughter died in the Cocoanut Grove fire. The man, who visualized his daughter in a telephone booth calling for him, became so preoccupied that he was often oblivious to his surroundings. The grieving person frequently expresses concern over this aspect of the grief reaction, fearing that such a response indicates approaching insanity.

Feelings of guilt compose yet another of the classes of symptoms of normal grief. The mourner often accuses himself of negligence and exaggerates thoughts, feelings, or actions toward the deceased which are other than positive. He frequently views himself as having failed the other, often expressing his failure in statements such as "If I had only . . . ."

Hostile reactions are also a component of the normal grieving process. The bereaved find themselves concerned about the irritability, anger, and loss of warmth they feel toward others. Lindemann noted that the bereaved may make great efforts to handle these feelings of hostility, often in a formalized and stiff manner of social interaction.

The final general class of symptoms of normal grief has to do with loss of patterns of conduct. For example, the bereaved person is often unable to initiate or maintain organized patterns of activity and instead may be restless or move about aimlessly. There seems to be a loss of zest, and tasks and activities are carried on as though with great effort. In addition the bereaved may discover that a large part of the activity which he formerly carried on in the company of the deceased has lost its significance, particularly habits of social interaction such as meeting friends, making conversation, and sharing projects or enterprises. For this reason the bereaved often becomes strongly dependent upon whoever stimulates him to activity and serves as an initiating agent.

Lindemann identified a sixth category of symptoms, which border on the pathological, in which traits of the deceased appear in the behavior of the bereaved. The traits of the deceased most likely to become evident in the mourner are symptoms shown during an illness preceding the death or behavior or personality traits which may have been shown prior to it.

Morbid Grief Reactions
In addition to these general classes of symptoms of normal grief, morbid grief reactions were also identified by Lindemann. The first category, delay of reaction, was found to be the most common and the most dramatic. The postponement may be brief or prolonged for a period of years. This type of response usually occurs if the death takes place at a time when the bereaved is confronted with important tasks or with the necessity for maintaining the morale of others. Distorted reactions comprise the second category and can be listed briefly:

Excessive activity with no sense of loss
Development of symptoms similar to those experienced
  by the deceased

Medical illness, psychosomatic in nature, developed in a
   close time relationship to the loss of an important person
Continued and progressive social isolation with alteration
   in relationships to friends and relatives
Extreme hostility against specific persons somehow
   connected with the death event
"Schizophrenic"-like wooden and formal conduct which
   masks the hostile feelings
Lasting change in former patterns of social interaction
Activities detrimental to one's own social and economic
   existence
Agitated depression

Successful Grieving

It was George Engel [5] who built upon Lindemann's work
to identify a process of grief work as necessary to successful
grieving. Grief work, or the work of mourning, can be identified as emancipation from bondage to the deceased, readjustment to the environment in which the deceased is missing,
and formation of new relationships. Successful grieving
consists of three phases: shock and disbelief, developing
awareness, and restitution or resolution.

   The first phase, shock and disbelief, can be characterized
as the "Oh no!" stage. The need to deny the loss is para-
mount, and the resulting behavior or style of loss denial
may run the gamut from verbal denial through incapacita-
tion. Each individual has his own style of denial, which is
determined partly by cultural factors and partly by previous
experiences with loss and separation. This phase is summa-
rized by Engel: "Distinctive of this initial phase are attempts

at protection against the effects of the overwhelming stress by raising the threshold against its recognition or against the painful feeling evoked thereby" [5].

Reality begins to assert itself in the second phase — developing awareness — which may begin very soon after the bereavement or may take some time to develop. It is at this time that awareness of the loss becomes acute. Crying frequently takes place as does anger toward the dead person for his desertion, displaced onto others or onto the self through self-injury or self-destructive behavior.

Restitution — the third phase — completes the work of mourning. Early in this period the memory of the dead person is elevated to a degree of perfection to the extent that realistic facets of the dead person's personality or behavior — if negative or socially unacceptable — may be overlooked. It may take many months for the mourner to be able to take a more realistic view of the deceased. For example, shortly after the assassinations of President John F. Kennedy and Senator Robert Kennedy a number of books and articles extolling their virtues were published. These publications were generally one-sided in that they overlooked less positive or socially unacceptable behavior and personality characteristics. However, after the passage of time, publications concerning the Kennedys began to present the total picture more accurately.

Aiding the Grieving Process

Mourning is frequently completed within the year following the death. However, when the mourner has not experienced all three phases of grieving, grieving cannot be said to have been completed nor can the work of mourning be finished. Unresolved grief can be the prelude to psychopathological depression requiring psychiatric treatment. For these reasons it becomes important that bereaved persons be helped to resolve their grief. Not until the work of mourning is completed can the work of living continue.

Anticipatory Grieving

The death of a loved one is a crisis and is therefore of concern to theoreticians and clinicians whose interest is crisis intervention and preventive psychiatry. Consistent with such a focus, a technique of preventive intervention called *anticipatory guidance* has been suggested by Gerald Caplan [2] as helpful in adjusting to the impact of loss. The primary intent of anticipatory guidance is to help persons to cope through discussion of the details of the impending crisis and through problem-solving before the crisis event occurs. Preventive intervention of this nature is most useful when it is not restricted to those awaiting crisis but is also available to those who will serve as helping persons. In addition to helping families of dying patients and staff members in coping with the crisis of death, anticipatory guidance also lays the foundation for effective grief work.

However, when mourning begins long before the death, families may finish grieving before the patient dies. Glaser and Strauss [7] caution that family members may not be able to help during the last stages of dying if, with too much advance warning, they prepare themselves so well that they give up the patient before he dies.

Ambivalence may be experienced by family members

who complete their grief work before the patient dies. They may feel resentful about the time and effort spent in visiting the dying patient and the money spent on hospital care. They often find themselves wishing they could go on with their own living, other interests, jobs, friends. Such feelings of hostility often provoke feelings of guilt.

Hospital staff members who are aware that anticipatory grieving is taking place will find it easier to be supportive of the family rather than to feel negatively toward relatives whom they perceive as rejecting. When staff members can be accepting of ambivalence, hostility, and feelings of guilt, they will be more open to therapeutic interaction and more helpful in the maintenance of mental health and the prevention of mental illness. It can be supportive for relatives to know that such feelings are normal components of grief work.

Weisman and Hackett [10] have identified a related phenomenon they call *premortem dying,* which may occur in the interactions between the dying patient and his family and may indicate that anticipatory grieving is taking place. The dying person is less and less often allowed to participate in decisions regarding the family or his own interests. Instead, family members frequently respond with "Don't you worry" and "Everything is being taken care of" to the dying person's questions about what is happening outside the hospital. It is not unusual to observe this phenomenon when dying is prolonged. While family members generally perceive their behavior as protecting the dying person from participating in stressful situations, such behavior does indicate a change in the family system and may indicate that they already think of him as no longer a part of the family.

When family members begin to take on the roles previously held by the dying person and exclude him from the family system, it may be difficult if not impossible for the dying person to re-enter the family system if he should recover. Only recently the wife of a patient with chronic glomerulonephritis told of her five-year experience in caring for her ill husband. The wife was also a nurse and personally cared for her husband during his long and frequent hospitalizations. Eventually, she began to assume the role of nurturer, provider, and decision-maker. After her husband had undergone a successful kidney transplantation and was able to resume his job, she found it impossible to give up or alter the roles she had taken on during his illness. He expected to take over the decision-making again, while she resumed the dependent role she had had during their courtship and early marriage. What happened was that this woman had finished her grieving and had become, in many ways, a different person. They were unable to resolve their interpersonal difficulties and are in the process of divorce.

The Three Phases of Successful Mourning

Specifically what can nurses do to assist the bereaved to successfully complete the work of mourning? It is during the first two phases of grieving — shock and disbelief and developing awareness — that health care personnel in institutional settings have most of their contact with grieving family members and friends. The nurse must recognize the normal grief pattern and not interfere with its course so that grieving can be successfully completed.

Behavior in the shock and disbelief phase reflects attempts by the bereaved to protect themselves either against recognition of the event or against the painful feeling it evokes. How individuals respond seems to be affected by their capacity for establishing meaningful relationships as well as by cultural factors. While some persons deny the event or refuse to believe that it occurred, others may protect themselves from the painful feeling evoked by the stress and may move to comfort those less close to the deceased in their grief. It is important in this phase to be guided by the knowledge that the mental mechanism of denial serves a therapeutic purpose in protecting the bereaved from painful knowledge with which he may be unable to cope. Aronson [1] suggests that persons be permitted to keep up the role important to them to the extent that this is possible. Lengthy maintenance of denial in the face of reality, however, signals distress. Resolution of grief cannot be achieved until the bereaved successfully completes each stage of mourning, and continuing denial prevents the mourner from moving on to the stage of developing awareness. A therapeutic maneuver which may be helpful in assisting an individual to move through this stage of the mourning process is the presentation of reality. The nurse expresses his or her own perceptions of the facts in the situation but avoids arguments based on logic, in the hope of encouraging the bereaved individual to move on to the stage of developing awareness.

During this second stage of mourning crying is one of the most evident activities. Because tears are a vital and important part of the process of normal grieving, they should not be discouraged and should be allowed to continue. On the other hand, while nurses should not be afraid to shed tears nor to see them shed, they may have contact with family members who do not cry as expected. Family members may be unable to cry either because of hostility or ambivalence toward the dead person or perhaps because they have already engaged in the process of premortem dying and have completed their grief work. Refusal to cry may be viewed as a protective mechanism that prevents the release of emotions, and persons who do not cry should not be viewed as heartless and inhuman. Encouraging persons to cry or otherwise to express emotion, when in fact they are unable to do so, increases their guilt, which in itself is a component of most grief reactions.

When mourners are able to, however, it is usually found helpful to allow them to express their emotions. In many instances health personnel move too quickly to suppress the expression of emotion, often through offering medication with a sedative effect. While some medication may be useful initially, overmedication only delays and prolongs the grieving process. We need to be more cautious about giving medication to bereaved persons and consider whether it will facilitate or subvert the grieving process.

During these two phases nurses usually are present to assist relatives in their bereavement. Such assistance requires the nurse to be a good listener who understands that time spent in hearing expressions of grief, recall of memories, and reminiscences will be very helpful in encouraging normal and successful grieving. This assists persons in the movement toward the third phase of mourning — restitution.

Restitution is assisted by the traditional religious mourning practices of the wake, the funeral, and expressions of condolence by friends. Today we seldom see the emotionalism, the retention of keepsakes like locks of hair, and the plumed hearses of the Victorian era, although they all provided a relief far beyond that given by stiff upper lips and the requests for no mourning and no flowers.

A recent exception occurred when the entire nation was assisted in its mourning following the death of President John F. Kennedy. People mourned in their living rooms in front of the television set, responding to the funeral dirge and the beat of the drum, reacting to the riderless horse and the draped hearse. The nation became actively involved in the burying of the dead. Institutionalization of the mourning experience in terms of the associated rituals helps to complete grief work [5]. Not only is the reality of death emphasized, but the rituals themselves allow for supportive interpersonal interaction to occur.

Another very public example is the way in which, after the assassination of Robert Kennedy, his family demonstrated coping with grief. The adults rallied around the children in a variety of ways. When adult family members were unable to meet the needs of the children, adults other than family members — John Glenn, for example — took over. Such flexibility of role function ensured that nurturing and control needs were met. In addition the three eldest children participated in the vigil at the hospital as well as in every aspect of the funeral ritual including bringing the coffin to New York City and the day of public mourning in Saint Patrick's Cathedral. They were joined at the funeral Mass by all the youngest, down to Douglas, who was then fourteen months old, where some of the older children participated as acolytes and assisted in bringing the bread and wine to the high altar. The entire family made the journey together on the train to Washington, D.C., and Arlington National Cemetery. In a discussion of the way in which Senator Kennedy's family participated in these events Gerald Caplan [3] notes the comfort and steadfast support the children received through their involvement as well as its positive influence upon the grieving process. He believes that through understanding the behavior of the Kennedy family we can learn to help others cope with the death of a parent or a significant person.

Further Considerations
Caplan [2] suggests still another helpful approach to the completion of successful grieving:

The hazards of mourning would also be reduced if the bereaved person were freed for a period from the demands of his job so that he could devote his energies to his "grief work." The possibility is suggested that public education and modification in industry might lead to the widespread adoption of the practice of offering "mourning leave" with pay, analogous to "sick leave."

Since the health care delivery system is one of the biggest businesses in the United States, its adoption of such a practice would constitute positive movement in the direction of mental health by those having the greatest interest in improving and preserving the health of the public.

It is seldom recognized that those who care for the dying

may also need to mourn the loss of a patient and work through their grief. Nurses may need a respite from hospital units, such as intensive care, where death often occurs. Periodic assignments to units where patients have high recovery rates and where the nurses' emotional investment may not be so prolonged might provide the opportunity.

Nursing educators must provide a means for nursing students to learn about grief and acquire the skills necessary to resolve their own grief and help others toward resolution. Nursing administrators need to ask for appropriate budgetary allowances which would make possible the provision of in-service programs designed to help nurses become grief facilitators. Clinical specialists in psychiatric nursing can also help individual nurses face problems squarely and serve as consultants to them in formulating a plan of care that would allow for grief work.

Recently it has been suggested that advantage be taken of the continuing march of technology which makes the sustaining of vital processes possible for increasingly longer periods of time. One suggestion has been to maintain persons defined as dead on machines capable of sustaining the bodily functions necessary to using organs for transplant purposes. Gaylin [6] suggests "wholesale and systematic salvage of useful body parts." He further suggests that

We could develop hospitals (an inappropriate word because it suggests the presence of living human beings), banks, or farms of cadavers which require feeding and maintenance, in order to be harvested. To the uninitiated the "new cadavers" in their rows of respirators would seem indistinguishable from comatose patients now residing in wards of chronic neurological hospitals.

These "new cadavers," which Gaylin renames "neomorts," could also be used, he suggests, to train medical students in physical examination and interns and residents in more difficult diagnostic procedures such as lumbar puncture, arteriogram, eye operations, skin grafts, and organ transplant. He suggests their further use as subjects in research on drug toxicity and experimental operative and diagnostic techniques. The possibilities, according to Gaylin, are limitless.

The obvious arguments for and against implementation of Gaylin's suggestions are likely to revolve around the question of humanitarianism, with the proponents arguing the promise of cure and eventual reduction of suffering and maintenance of life, while the opponents argue that such measures are inhumane. Strong opposition is likely to come also from persons who demand the right to be allowed to die with dignity [9].

Another factor should be considered in the debate. This factor is the effect that such technological maintenance of organs would have upon the ability of the bereaved to resolve their grief through successful completion of each of the three stages of grieving. Would it be possible to resolve grief with the knowledge that the body of the person for whom one is grieving is being maintained elsewhere and used for medical research purposes? It is vital to consider the effects of such measures on the living as well as on the dying.

Proper management of the grieving response may prevent prolonged and serious alterations in the social adjustment of the bereaved as well as potential physiologically and emotionally pathological states. It is obvious that dying patients, their families and friends, and their nurses can be helped through the crisis of death and the process of bereavement. What is required is an intellectual and emotional understanding of the mourning process and of distortions of grief reactions, the delivery and acceptance of support and comfort, and a knowledge of how to cope with the pain bereavement brings.

References

1. Aronson, G. J. Treatment of the Dying Person. In Feifel, H. (Ed.), *The Meaning of Death*. New York: McGraw-Hill, 1959, pp. 35–36.
2. Caplan, G. *Principles of Preventive Psychiatry*. New York: Basic Books, 1964.
3. Caplan, G., with Cadden, V. Lessons in bravery. *McCall's* 95: 85, 1968.
4. Cobb, S., and Lindemann, E. Neuropsychiatric observations after the Cocoanut Grove fire. *Ann. Surg.* 117:814, 1943.
5. Engel, G. *Psychological Development in Health and Disease*. Philadelphia: Saunders, 1962.
6. Gaylin, W. Harvesting the dead: The potential for recycling human bodies. *Harper's* 249:23, 1974.
7. Glaser, B. G., and Strauss, A. L. *Awareness of Dying*. Chicago: Aldine, 1965.
8. Lindemann, E. Symptomatology and management of acute grief. *Am. J. Psychiatry* 101:141, 1944.
9. Mannes, M. *Last Rights*. New York: Morrow, 1974.
10. Weisman, A. D., and Hackett, T. P. Predilection to death: Death and dying as a psychiatric problem. *Psychosom. Med.* 23:232, 1961.

3. IF YOU WERE DYING...

Ruth A. Assell

If you were dying.... Imagine for a moment what this really means. Your own death. A sobering and perhaps a lonely thought. With the contemplation of death come thoughts of what life means: family, friends, work, talents, potentials, accomplishments, failures, and beliefs about life after death. These are all aspects of what it means to die.

Reflection on one's own death can produce numerous reactions, among them fear, guilt, sadness, peace, panic, grief, and anxiety. For many the predominant feeling such reflection elicits is that of unreality — an unconscious belief in one's own immortality. To some extent an individual extends this feeling of immortality to his family and close friends. Since no one has yet discovered the key to immortality, each of us is faced with the prospect of dying. This fact remains despite the various ordinary and extraordinary techniques that have been developed to prolong life or, rather, postpone death. Dying is one life task that each individual must perform entirely for himself. This is not to say that he must die alone. Those around the dying person should realize that he is not devoid of memories, desires, and hopes for recovery and for life after death, and that he is affected by his internal and external environment. Much too often, however, a person is not allowed to die with that human dignity consistent with his identity and individuality.

One purpose of this chapter is to attempt to define the fine line between isolation and abandonment on the one hand and overcompensation for professional and personal fallibility on the other. It is my belief that the prime purpose, goal, and direction of care of the dying person and his family is to ensure with whatever measures are appropriate the right of the person to die with dignity, identity, and individuality and the right of the family to consideration, support, and empathy.

Since, although perhaps unconsciously, a person's philosophy of death and dying is closely patterned on his philosophy of life and living, it behooves the nurse not only to ascertain the philosophy of the dying person and his family but also to identify her own beliefs, attitudes, and feelings in this regard. Being aware of differing philosophies of life and death is essential for the nurse caring for the dying person [1, 2, 6, 7]. Ignorance in this regard can hinder the nurse's ability to cope, and to assist the dying person and his family to cope, with the realities of dying.

In addition to being prepared to understand a particular patient's philosophy of life and death, the nurse, to be of assistance to the dying person and his family, must attempt to know them as people. Because death is such a very personal experience, it is the responsibility of the nurse to know the person of the patient. She or he must attempt to learn and be open to the patient's likes and dislikes; role in his family and community; concerns and fears; hopes and desires; need to love and be loved; need to trust and be trusted; need not to be shunned and isolated; need for physical, psychological, spiritual, and social comfort; and finally need to be seen and treated as a person rather than merely as the object of many ministrations.

There are numerous ways to elicit such information. The most direct, but not always the easiest, is to talk with the person and his family; to listen not only to what is said but also to what is meant. The nurse thus becomes involved.

Involvement — that once forbidden condition that if indulged in by a nurse stripped her of what was commonly referred to as professionalism. In addition to the risk of being labeled unprofessional by colleagues, the nurse who allows herself to become involved with the dying person and his family runs an additional risk: that of being hurt by the death of a person who has come to be a meaningful part of her life. Many a nurse is not ready, willing, or able to cope with this type of grief. This is all right, but she must also realize why it is that she does not choose to become involved with the dying person. She must not simply hide behind the guise of professionalism. These may seem like harsh words, but assigning a nurse who cannot deal with the concept and reality of death and dying to care for a dying person is somewhat analogous to assigning a nurse who cannot deal with abortions to the care of a person who has presented herself at a hospital for an abortion.

It might be helpful for the nurse caught in the dilemma of indecision regarding involvement or not to reflect again on the phrase "If I were dying . . . ." Does the meaning of involvement become clear when viewed from this point of reference? Would a nurse or caring person who showed in some way that he was involved be meaningful to you if you were dying? Would you prefer a nurse who could cope or help you to cope with the reality of your own death? Now, consider for a moment the elderly man in Room 415 or the young mother in Room 612 or the teenager attending the hematology clinic. What does involvement mean to them? Granted, involvement to the point of immobility is of benefit to no one: neither nurse, dying person, nor family. Fear of this occurring, however, must not stop the nurse from caring and showing it. It is far more tragic to be stopped by fear of emotional involvement than it is to attempt to prevent one more person from dying in isolation.

The Nurse and the Dying Patient: Interaction?
The jacket of the book *Awareness of Dying* by Glaser and Strauss [3] illustrates well a common phenomenon observed in the care of the dying person. The jacket shows three people: a dying patient, a doctor, and a nurse. The dying patient is depicted as seeing no evil; the doctor as hearing no evil; and the nurse as speaking no evil. The first page of the book contains an anecdote.

Once upon a time a patient died and went to heaven, but was not certain where he was. Puzzled, he asked a nurse who was standing near by: "Nurse, am I dead?" She replied: "Have you asked your doctor?"

This story tells a tale that is all too familiar to most nurses. The name of the game is: Don't let the dying person know what is happening to him.

Nurses' Reluctance to Face Death
The dynamics of the nurse—dying person interaction are one aspect of nursing care of the dying which deserves special attention. By virtue of the commitment of her role the nurse is in a key position to assist the dying person to perform his final act with dignity and integrity. She is in a position to offer the support and assistance that are

necessary to him and his family over a period of time. Generally when a person enters a hospital as a patient, the focus of the patient, family, and staff is on recovery, preserving life, getting well. As long as a chance for recovery exists, the medical and nursing staff are able to comfort themselves with the notion that they are using all their knowledge and skill to heal. This attitude is understandable, since the nursing and medical educational process is geared toward healing. Assisting an individual to regain or maintain his potential for health is one way that staff can fulfill themselves and their potential.

As a result of this recovery orientation a conflict often arises when the stage of hoping for recovery passes and it becomes obvious that the person is going to die. The death of a person is not a desired outcome of nursing care. Death is more often than not seen as a personal failure on the part of the health care team. Nursing education does not, for the most part, prepare nurses to deal with death and the dying person. As recently as five to seven years ago many nursing curricula, if they dealt with death at all, limited their considerations to postmortem care. Death is a reality and an aspect of life which nurses must deal with, however, if the goal of total comprehensive patient care is to be achieved [5]. For the sake of the dying person and his family, nurses must come to grips with death and dying.

Patient's Level of Awareness

The terminally ill or dying person experiences several levels of awareness regarding his condition (as discussed in Chapter 1). First, he may be unaware of his prognosis; second, he may suspect that he is dying; third, he may know with certainty that he is dying [3]. In this chapter these three levels of patient awareness will be explored only as they directly relate to the nursing care that is provided. Provision of nursing care will be discussed from the point of view of the nurse who has already reached the third level of awareness regarding any particular patient. In other words, the nurse knows with certainty that the patient is dying.

Provision of comprehensive care to the dying person who is totally unaware of his impending death (that is, in a *closed-awareness context*) can be a serious predicament for the nurse. One difficulty arises out of a conflict grounded in the "right to be told" philosophy of care. The nurse may feel strongly that to allow the dying person to remain unaware of his impending death is wrong. She may feel that the patient has the right to know his fate, so that he can prepare himself for death. Her dilemma arises from the fact that she is limited in what information she can divulge to the dying patient and his family. In most institutions it is still the physician's prerogative to determine whether or not the dying person should be told.

This state of patient unawareness can be quite stressful for the nurse. The nurse-patient relationship begins quickly to resemble a fencing match with the appropriate warning issued: "on guard." The nurse must be constantly on guard not to let the truth slip. One of her nursing goals is to make the dying person as comfortable as possible, but this must be accomplished in such a way as not to arouse the patient's suspicions. Caught in this stressful circumstance, just how comforting can the nurse be? She is placed in continuous intimate contact with the dying person without being given the right to do what she thinks is best for him. If the nurse is to provide the most appropriate care for the dying patient and his family, she must be allowed (in fact, expected) to participate in the decisions which determine her action regarding the emotional and physical support surrounding his care.

An even more difficult problem for many nurses is the provision of nursing care to the patient who suspects that his illness is terminal — that he is going to die. This creates a *suspicion context*. The stresses of the *closed-awareness* state are now multiplied. The dying person more than likely begins to search for cues and clues which will either confirm or refute his suspicions. The logical target for his queries is the nurse or nurse's aide. These are the people who, by virtue of their role and function, have the most intimate contact with the patient.

Nurses handle the suspicious person in a variety of ways depending on, first, how comfortable they themselves are with death and dying and, second, how obligated they feel to continue the "keep the patient in the dark" game. These methods of patient management are well-known tricks of the trade. They have been around so long that they border on tradition and are passed from one generation to the next as surely as a poor teacher's reputation is passed from class to class.

Because the dying person is not aware of the sacredness of the topic about which he is seeking information, he may do the unforgivable thing — he may approach the matter head on. How does the nurse handle the question "Nurse, am I going to die?" Guided by tradition she might respond, "Have you asked your doctor?" or "I'm sorry, I can't discuss this with you, you'll have to speak with your doctor." Another method of fielding such a question is to change the subject: "Die? Don't be silly. It's such a beautiful day. Would you like the radio on?" Often the change of subject is followed by a rather speedy departure from the patient and the room. Some nurses deal best with the direct question by pretending that they never heard it; others by "hearing" a call for help from the room across the hall. Their exit is often accompanied by a trailing voice promising to be "right back." Many times the nurse does not return but sends someone else in her stead. If the dying person does not learn the game rules quickly but continues to question the staff about his condition, he may find himself the "forgotten man." His physical needs are not neglected, but they are met in the most expeditious way. An air of business surrounds the task, with perhaps a running commentary describing all the things to be done, all the patients to be cared for, and a hurried "I'm sorry that I can't spend more time with you."

The responses mentioned thus far are not really satisfying for either the dying person or the nurse. The patient will continue his inquiries and the nurse will become frustrated, frightened, and guilty. More appropriate responses and actions on the part of the nurse when asked this awesome question might be the following:

"Do you feel you are going to die?"
"What makes you ask that question?"

"What makes you think you are dying?"
"Do you feel your illness is terminal?"

Appropriate actions include sitting down and allowing the
dying person to express his feelings, fears, and doubts about
his condition.

The question "Am I going to die?" often carries with it
the question "Why?" This is particularly true in the case
of a child or young adult. In such cases it is important for
the nurse to be ready to acknowledge to herself and the
dying person that there may not be answers, or at least
comforting answers, to some questions regarding the why
of death. Admitting to not having an answer may provide
more support to the dying person than grabbing for one of
the clichés that are often used at such times. Although a
ready command of all the answers is part of the traditional
professional image, it is not a very realistic expectation here.

Many times the dying person's questions regarding his
condition and future are his efforts to establish lines of
communication that will bring him into harmony with his
immediate surroundings. Questioning may be his attempt
to become a part of what is happening to him. The nurse
must be sensitive enough to determine the intent and real
meaning of the questions posed.

The responses suggested afford the dying person the
opportunity, if he wishes it, to explore aloud feelings, fears,
doubts, and concerns relative to his present and his immediate future. He may not be ready at that point actively to
pursue the topic of his own death, but he should be allowed
the choice, the human freedom, to decide. The right

response opens the door for further discussion, if and when he wants to pursue it. Although it may be difficult for the nurse to place herself in the vulnerable position of discussing death with a dying person, it is the right of the dying person to be given this choice. A direct response also indicates to the dying person something of the nurse's openness and concern. She is interested in him as an individual and is worthy of his trust. This knowledge on the part of the patient can, and in all likelihood will, be a source of support to him during the days preceding his death. Two of the most important services the nurse can provide the dying at this particular time are her sensitivity and her availability to him.

The third phase of awareness experienced by the dying person is that of a full realization that he is dying (*open awareness*). He may have reached this stage by accurately interpreting the seriousness of his symptoms or by adroitly sorting out cues that the nurse may have deliberately or unwittingly dropped; or his physician may have decided that now is the time to tell him that his case is terminal — that he is going to die. No matter what the source of information, the knowledge of the reality of his situation is often difficult for him to cope with. Grieving may begin. The dying person begins the process of mourning his own death.

This awareness of impending death may occur relatively close to the actual death of the individual. Once again, the nurse can be of great help to the patient and his family. It is during this third phase of awareness, more than any other, that the dying may feel the need to talk, not necessarily about his death but perhaps about phases of his life which are particularly meaningful to him. In order to cope with what is happening to him he may feel the need to review his life: his accomplishments, his failures, his joys, his disappointments. At this time he needs to be reassured that his life was, and therefore his death is, meaningful. One of the most painful, tragic, and disturbing experiences for a dying person is to believe that his life has had no impact on anything or anyone. If the dying person has a family and friends who are near, their help can be elicited. If he is alone, it falls to the nurse to assume this role. Supportive reassurance by family and nurse may be handled directly by allowing the dying person to verbalize what he considers to be his failures or mistakes in life. If he feels the need to express regret or sorrow for past occurrences, allow him to do so. Allowing the dying person to express regret does not permit a moral judgment on the part of the nurse. This is neither expected nor desirable. In fact to weigh the rightness or wrongness of the dying patient's past has no role in the provision of nursing care. The function the patient's "confession" does serve is the one already mentioned; it allows the dying person to express his feelings about a life past, to right things in his own mind.

In addition to the support which the nurse and family can provide, solace may often be given to the dying person by his spiritual director or the hospital chaplain. This option should be provided with the nurse or family making the necessary arrangements according to the patient's wishes. The dying person has the right to the comforts provided by his professed religion. On the other hand, if he does not

wish to speak with a representative of a church or a religion,
it does not fall within the nurse's role to coerce him to do so.

The Nurse and the Dying Patient: Intervention
In addition to allowing or assisting the dying person to
attain an inner peace, the nurse should be actively trying
to maintain, as it were, an outer peace. This refers to ensur-
ing peace and integrity within the patient's hospital environment. In some instances the nurse can see to this herself;
sometimes she must rely on the help and understanding of
others such as the family, physician, other staff, and hospital administration. Thus, one of her roles is to be an
advocate for the rights of this dying person. The actions
necessary to assure the peace and integrity of the environment include, in part, the following.

*First: The nurse should make herself available to the dying
person.*

Availability, as used here, includes not only physical
presence but also a sensitivity to patient need. The nurse
must realize when the dying person needs someone physically present and when he needs to be alone. The nurse
must be honest enough with herself, however, not to confuse allowing the dying person to be alone with not wanting
to enter his room. It is so easy to say, "I'm in the way. He
really wants to be by himself to think things through."
The nurse must also be on guard not to confuse the dying
person's silence with his wanting to be alone. The first does
not necessarily follow from the second. He may not want

to talk, but he may want and need the physical presence of someone whom he trusts. He may have the need to know someone does care and is aware that he is experiencing many emotions which he cannot as yet verbalize. He may want someone close who he feels understands that he is facing the beginning of a very difficult life task.

Second: The nurse should make provision for significant others to be with the dying person.

A person goes through life surrounded by other people whom he considers close. He cannot think of the past, or for that matter the future, without thinking of the people who have played an important role in his life. For this reason a comfort that should be afforded every dying person is provision for the significant persons in his life to be with him if he so chooses. This may mean allowing relatives, friends, children, grandchildren, and so forth to visit and be with him. The hospitalization, in and of itself, has stripped this person of much of his identity. It has removed him from the environment with which he is familiar. It has effectively removed him from the significant others in his life. If hospitals and the professionals in them have been responsible for so effectively isolating the patient, is there any reason why these same hospitals and professionals cannot take the necessary steps to reinstate him socially?

Hospital policies, with few exceptions, restrict visitors by age, number of people, and time. Reasons for these rules are a whole issue in themselves. The question here is: Are these policies so rigidly guarded, so sacred, that they cannot be altered or waived in the interest of the dying person and his family? Are the rules more sacred than the persons they were meant to serve? If seeing and being with their children will ease the pain and loss for a young mother or father who is dying, why not allow it? If a man has spent his whole life surrounded by friends and family, why deprive him of their companionship now? If one of the nurse's primary responsibilities is to ensure the dying person's right to die with the dignity consistent with his identity and individuality, why let him die with only the hum of the respirator or the bleep of the monitor to comfort him?

Third: The nurse should make an effort to surround the dying person with those things that are familiar, habitual, or of value to him.

Simple, everyday things which are so much a part of life that they are taken for granted are often abruptly eliminated from the patient's life by the normal hospital routine. Examples include food, drink, clothing, and personal items. Consideration should be given to the culture, custom, and life style that have surrounded the person since birth. For example, if having a glass of wine with the meal has been a custom, why not allow the family or hospital to provide this? Surely such a simple comfort cannot be disruptive.

The difficulty and possible senselessness of going against a patient's long-ingrained habits are illustrated by the case of Mrs. E., a 103-year-old resident of a nursing home, whose diagnosis was arteriosclerotic heart disease. Mrs. E.'s greatest comfort and joy in life was bread, butter, and jam sandwiches. She preferred these sandwiches to the exclusion of practically anything else. Mrs. E. would beg the aides, staff, or anyone she could corner to bring her bread, butter, and jam in place of her regular meals. Sometimes she succeeded. The nursing staff were horrified. Mrs. E. was not getting a well-balanced diet. A full-scale program was launched to see that Mrs. E. ate meat, potatoes, vegetables, and salad — the recommended nutritional basic four. Mrs. E. was not at all impressed with this program of care. She would bribe, sneak, beg, and cry for bread, butter, and jam, often to no avail.

Looking at the situation objectively, one should commend the staff on their efforts to provide this 103-year-old woman with a well-balanced diet. Viewing it subjectively, one might ask, why? Why should this woman be deprived of the one joy she had left in life? Why should she be forced into the antics characteristic of childhood — begging, sneaking, and being made to feel guilty about her behavior? It is difficult to believe that the therapeutic management carried out outweighed the comfort and preservation of dignity and self-worth that a relaxation of the rules would have provided for this individual.

Many more examples could be cited to demonstrate this point. Every nurse comes across similar situations each day. Perhaps the individual nurse is not in a position to correct every situation she encounters, but she *is* in a position to try — to act as patient advocate in the hospital setting.

*Fourth: The nurse should give the dying person an oppor-
tunity to put his life in order.*

If the person desires, the nurse should assist him in making provisions for the drawing of a will. He should be
allowed to advise his family on their future needs and assist
them in planning for the future. He should be given the
opportunity to settle his debts. Last, but not least, he
should be assisted in securing the kind of spiritual assistance
he deems necessary.

The Dying Comatose Patient

The majority of comments thus far have dealt with the
dying person who is consciously aware of what is happening to and around him. Attention will now be turned to
the dying comatose person. What supportive care can the
nurse provide him? The focus of nursing care in this situation is primarily on physical support to the dying person
and emotional and psychosocial support to the family.

For many nurses care of the dying comatose patient does
not provide the problem nor the threat that care of the
conscious person does. The whole dilemma of talking to
the person about dying and its meaning to him is eliminated.
All efforts and energies can now be most appropriately
directed toward providing comfort. The lack of sensory
response on the part of the comatose person does not, however, relieve the nurse of the task of providing emotional,
social, and physical comfort. Despite his apparent oblivi-
ousness of the persons and things that surround him, he
should be communicated with verbally and through touch.

It is still of the utmost importance that the patient have the feeling that the nurse is there, is concerned, and wants to help in whatever way she can.

The nurse should be extremely careful not to speak about the dying comatose person "over" him. In spite of knowing that unconscious patients may be able to hear although they cannot respond, staff are often guilty of conversing with each other or with family members in the presence of the comatose person, as if he were not there. The nurse, in addition to being aware of this pitfall herself, can assist the family in defining their role with the dying patient. She can encourage them to talk *to*, not about or over the dying family member. Not only does such an activity help to preserve the dignity of the patient, it also relieves the family, to some extent, of a feeling of helplessness. Encouraging the family to talk to their dying comatose relative serves the additional function of giving the family an opportunity to disengage from him gradually rather than abruptly.

The Family and the Dying Patient

Now try to put yourself in the place of the family of the dying person: "If I were that family member . . . ." The family's role in the care of the dying person is, or should be, a significant one. The family is one of the nurse's best resources in the planning and implementation of total care for the dying person. After the patient himself, or if the patient cannot communicate, they are the best suited to identify the patient's needs. They should be encouraged to participate in the planning and implementation of care whenever and however feasible.

The family is important as one of the chief supports of
the dying person as he embarks on and eventually completes the life task of dying. If the family members are to
support the dying person, they in turn must be supported.
The role of the nurse should include this function, since
she is the person who has, or should have, the closest relationship with both the dying person and his family. How
can the nurse best support the family? Many ways exist.

First: The nurse should talk with and listen to the family.

Allow the family members to express both their positive
and negative feelings about the dying person. This requires
time and a suitable place. The family should be allowed to
begin to mourn the loss of one of its members. They should
be allowed to express sorrow or guilt; relief or frustration;
and love, ambivalence, or hate without having a moral judgment placed on the feelings they express. (The nurse may
be instrumental in assisting the family to explore and work
through some of these feelings, or she may prefer to refer
them to someone else.)

*Second: The family should not be isolated from the foci
of care.*

Family members should be allowed to participate actively
in caring for the patient if they so desire, rather than being
sent from the room each time a nursing or medical task is
performed. Rules, regulations, and policies that tend to
isolate the family should be carefully scrutinized and revised

as necessary. Care should be taken not to relegate the family to a waiting room down at the end of the hallway, where chances of direct contact or confrontation with nursing and medical personnel are minimized.

Third: The nurse should assist the family to talk to the dying patient about his death.

More often than not, family members also use avoidance, denial, or isolation techniques in their approach to the dying person. If the nurse has worked through her own feelings and is aware of the dying person's needs, she can help the family approach the situation in a way that is beneficial to both the dying person and the family.

Fourth: The nurse should let the family know that she is concerned about them and their dying family member.

One way of letting the family know she is concerned for them is by encouraging family expression and participation, as already discussed. Furthermore at the time of death it is not inappropriate for the nurse to cry. It may be most natural and comforting for both her and the family. The knowledge that the death of a loved one means something to the nurse is meaningful and comforting to the family. Sorrow expressed over the loss caused by death is not the right of the family alone.

The family does need support, understanding, and empathy at this time of crisis. They are often physically as well as emotionally exhausted, particularly if the terminal illness has been a lingering one. They probably have been racing back and forth between hospital and home. If the medical facility is located in a large city, some distance from their home, they may have had to leave other family members and responsibilities to be near the dying family member.

If a lack of respect and consideration is shown the family of the dying person by hospital staff, this is often not as calculated as it appears. The staff may be so caught up in the importance of their own role and the service they are providing that they actually forget that this dying patient has a family — a family who is concerned, worried, grief-stricken, and just plain tired. Perhaps if the staff would stop to think for a moment how they would want to be treated if they were in the family's shoes, attitudes would change.

Little things such as offering coffee or a cold drink; providing a comfortable chair; taking a moment, several times in the day and night, to talk with the family about the dying person's condition all go a long way toward making the family a part of what is happening. If the family are strange to the city, suggesting places to eat or to wait, such as parks, might help to relieve the tension of the vigil for them.

Many other little considerations could be enumerated, but the best advice and perhaps the key to the situation is to imagine, If I were that family member . . . .

The Dying Person: Home Care
Up to this point the focus has been on nursing care of the dying person and his family within the hospital setting.

To complete the picture, consideration should be given to the care of the dying person and his family in the home setting. Not all deaths occur within the hospital setting; many persons still do die at home. Furthermore many of the persons who die in hospitals or similar institutions begin the process of dying before hospitalization. Community health nurses are faced daily with dying patients and their families. What is the community health nurse's role in assisting these individuals? All the points mentioned previously can be applied to the home setting. An additional consideration is the fact that within the home it is the client and family who maintain the power and control that in the hospital are relegated to the physicians and nurses. Besides providing the family with a slight advantage, family awareness of control also serves the even more important function of assisting the community health nurse in planning her care *with* rather than *for* this individual and his family. If she neglects to include these important persons in her planning and provision of care, her efforts to help will in most instances be futile or at best will fall short of the desired goal.

For the family and the dying person in the home situation, the community health nurse may be the only link to the medical profession and the provision of care. The physician directs the medical program, for the most part, by communicating with the community health nurse. It is she who assesses, manages, and evaluates the care of the dying person in the home setting. The family rely on her to guide the care of the dying family member. The community health nurse has to be very astute in determining how much responsibility the family can assume for the care of the patient. She must be extremely careful not to overwhelm the family members by heaping all the caring tasks on them.

The nursing role of supporting the family through this crisis of terminal illness and death takes on added dimensions when the dying person is cared for in the home. In this situation the family are forced by time and space to spend time with and around the dying family member. They cannot leave the dying person as they might if he were hospitalized. They are faced daily with the reality of the situation. They may have to deal with frustration and guilt if for their own well-being they must temporarily retreat from the situation. Many times this needed retreat from the home environment meets with disapproval from other relatives and neighbors. Because society is not as yet comfortable in coping with death and dying, it often places unrealistic expectations on the family of a dying person. It is society's belief that the family members must devote every minute, day and night, to the vigilant care of the dying relative [4]. They are expected to exhibit superhuman endurance in the face of this crisis situation. They must not participate in any activity which in any way gives them the appearance of being joyful, relaxed, or not constantly aware that one of their family is dying.

In the case of a dying elderly parent, the family member may be torn between his responsibilities to the parent and his responsibilities to his own family. Young children may not be able to understand why their normal routine has been altered since grandma became sick. They do not know why everyone whispers when grandma's illness is discussed. They may be confused, frustrated, and disturbed because everyone is so somber and sad. It is, indeed, a difficult time for the child — but it need not be so, if adults themselves can only cope more adequately with death and dying. The role of the community health nurse is to assist the entire family in attaining and maintaining a healthy adjustment to the crisis they are experiencing.

Whatever the circumstances, the family is placed under a great deal of stress and is in need of whatever support the nurse can provide. In addition to the ways already mentioned, the nurse can support the family members by allowing them to express their ambivalence toward the situation that has been imposed on them, and to express and work through their feelings so that they are better able to cope with it. The nurse may be instrumental in helping the family to realize the importance of meeting their own needs for rest and relaxation. She should emphasize that by allowing themselves this respite from constant vigilance they are not only maintaining their own health but in the long run are actually benefiting the dying person; that is, if they are rested and relaxed themselves, they will be better able to meet the needs of the dying family member. Just convincing the family of this is not enough, however. The nurse should also assist them in taking positive, concrete steps to find someone who can provide this needed relief. Homemaker or sitter service may allow for some respite from constant care.

Although caring for the dying person in the home may be more difficult for the family, it does provide distinct advantages and comfort to the dying person. He is not forced to assume the anonymity of the hospitalized patient, nor is he removed from what is familiar and comfortable to him. With the help of his family and the community health nurse, his individuality and integrity are more easily preserved.

A common concern and fear of family members is: What should we do when death is imminent? Should we call the rescue squad; rush the dying person to the hospital; or try to resuscitate him ourselves? Just what are we expected to do?

Preparation of the family for the moment of death should be an ongoing process, beginning with the time that all are aware that the illness is terminal. The physician and community health nurse should work closely with the family to help them devise a plan with which they are comfortable. If the family have come to grips with the terminal nature of the illness and have chosen to care for the dying person at home, then the best course of action would seem to be one that does not call for heroic measures of resuscitation. Arriving at this decision is probably one of the most difficult tasks the family will have to perform. They are in need of constant, continuous support and reassurance that their decision to allow their loved one to die without heroic measures is a wise and valid one.

The nurse may want to make herself physically available to the family at this time. She may encourage them to call her when they think death is imminent. If this is not possible, she should at least make provision to visit the family as soon as possible after death occurs.

For the dying person death is the end of the crisis: for

the family it may be only the beginning. After the death of a family member, the family is in need of continued empathy, support, and reassurance that they did the right things — that they did their best for the dying family member. Several visits by the community health nurse, after the funeral, are important in helping the family work through the grief process and readjust their family life styles.

Conclusion

The nurse, whether based in the hospital or in the community, has the responsibility to assist the dying person and his family to cope with this life task in such a way that the dignity, integrity, and individuality of each remain intact.

References

1. Assell, R. A. An existential approach to death. *Nurs. Forum* 8:200, 1969.
2. Feifel, H. (Ed.). *The Meaning of Death.* New York: McGraw-Hill, 1959.
3. Glaser, B. G., and Strauss, A. L. *Awareness of Dying.* Chicago: Aldine, 1965.
4. Human, M. E. Death of a neighbor. *Am. J. Nurs.* 73:1914, 1973.
5. Kavanaugh, R. E. Helping patients who are facing death. *Nursing '74* 4:35, 1974.
6. Marcel, G. *Being and Having.* New York: Harper & Row, 1949.
7. Sartre, J. P. *Being and Nothingness* (2nd ed.). New York: Citadel, 1965.

4. THE RIGHT TO DIE WITH DIGNITY

Clark Hopkins

In view of the increasing interest in and concern about this controversial issue, I should like to plead urgently the cause of the right to die with dignity and a minimum amount of pain, from the viewpoint of the patient rather than of the health professional. This is not a particularly cheerful subject, but it is a bright one compared with dying by slow and painful degrees.

Early Efforts to Establish the Right to Die
In 1970 I went to an Ann Arbor meeting on aging that was the first step toward the White House Conference on Aging the following year. The purpose of this first step was to reach people at the grass roots, to find out what the problems of aging were, and to ask for suggestions as to what might be done about them. What troubled me most was simply the threat that faced with a long, painful, terminal illness or mental deterioration I should be kept alive against my will. No one else had brought up the point that the life of the elderly came to an end, and when I voiced my concerns the group reacted with dismay and aversion. My motion was accepted that this problem be raised at the White House Conference and an appropriate solution sought; but when I requested that the group support a proposal granting to each individual the right to die with dignity, I was voted down by a large majority. Three from the small audience came up afterward, however, and told of close relatives or friends who had been kept alive far too long. They wished to support my stand, and they hoped that something might be done. (This has been my experience

each of the half dozen times that I have spoken in this cause. Although my motions have been solidly voted down, each time people with painful, bitter memories of close friends or relatives kept alive through endless, hopeless, painful days have expressed their steadfast support and the hope that some appropriate action may be taken.)

We all know of specific examples of people who have been miraculously brought back to health after long desperate illnesses, as well as of some who have been kept alive too long. I am not familiar with all aspects of the fatal and near-fatal sicknesses and diseases, but I am concerned, primarily and selfishly, with my own case: my right to die with dignity and a minimum amount of pain.

I should like to point out that there is a vast difference between the establishment of the right to die and the exercise of that right. I make no claim that, were this right established, I would exercise it. I am concerned, however, that the option exist.

The Living Will

A step in this direction has been taken by the Euthanasia Educational Council of New York. This society has phrased and made available a *Living Will,* a request for the cessation of heroic measures and even for the hastening of death under appropriate circumstances (Figure 1).

This request for an easy, kindly death (and it is a *request,* not a legally binding document) has been formulated to meet the new conditions brought about by the artificial means and heroic measures now available for prolonging

**TO MY FAMILY, MY PHYSICIAN, MY LAWYER, MY CLERGYMAN
TO ANY MEDICAL FACILITY IN WHOSE CARE I HAPPEN TO BE
TO ANY INDIVIDUAL WHO MAY BECOME RESPONSIBLE FOR
MY HEALTH, WELFARE OR AFFAIRS**

Death is as much a reality as birth, growth, maturity and old age—it is
the one certainty of life. If the time comes when I, _____
_____ can no longer take part
in decisions for my own future, let this statement stand as an expression
of my wishes, while I am still of sound mind.

If the situation should arise in which there is no reasonable expectation
of my recovery from physical or mental disability, I request that I be
allowed to die and not be kept alive by artificial means or "heroic
measures." I do not fear death itself as much as the indignities of
deterioration, dependence and hopeless pain. I, therefore, ask that
medication be mercifully administered to me to alleviate suffering even
though this may hasten the moment of death.

This request is made after careful consideration. I hope you who care
for me will feel morally bound to follow its mandate. I recognize that
this appears to place a heavy responsibility upon you, but it is with the
intention of relieving you of such responsibility and of placing it upon
myself in accordance with my strong convictions, that this statement
is made.

Signed _____

Date _____

Witness _____

Witness _____

Copies of this request have been given to _____

_____

_____

_____

_____

Figure 1. A *Living Will*, developed by the Euthanasia Educational
Council. Reprinted with permission of the Euthanasia Educational
Council, 250 West 57th St., New York, N. Y. 10019.

life far beyond what previously may have been called the normal span. It is assumed that all the new discoveries should serve not merely to keep the patient alive but to assist in his recovery so that, at least in part, life may become again a blessing — "something to be glad of," as my dictionary defines the word — rather than a burden.

The Move to Specialized Care

Previous to the new discoveries and the development of artificial means of prolonging life, there was an unprecedented increase in reliance on hospitals for care of the sick. Before the First World War the hospital was resorted to only in extreme emergencies. In New Haven where I lived as a child there was a very good hospital, good at any rate for that long ago day; but in a family of six children we all had measles and mumps at home, all the children were delivered at home by the family physician, and when I had scarlet fever I was put to bed and a sheet put over the door to keep the infection from spreading. When one of my brothers caught it he was put to bed beside me, and the rest of the family carried on as usual.

I point this out because it is not just the recent drugs and new machines that have revolutionized the care of the sick and the aged. Beginning with the First World War there has been a steady shift away from the family doctor to the specialist and the hospital for serious injuries and diseases; and the two together have given tremendous numbers of extra years, often happy ones, to tremendous numbers of people. Death, however, waits at the end, and just as there is no escape from death, so there is no avoidance, if one lives long enough, of physical and mental deterioration.

1971 White House Conference on Aging

In 1971 I was appointed a Michigan delegate to the White House Conference on Aging [5], and in Washington I made proposals that went a good deal beyond the recommendations of the Euthanasia Educational Council.* I had been assigned to the section "Spiritual Well-Being of the Aging," and my experience at the state level had taught me that any proposal to terminate the prolongation of a life, a prolongation which is being carried out by either natural or artificial means, would be turned down. Incidentally it is no easy task nowadays to distinguish between natural and artificial means. Natural means are food and fluids; artificial means are stimulants and intravenous feeding. On which side are oxygen, antibiotics, and pacemakers? These are taken for granted now, as digitalis and sulfa drugs were accepted long ago.

In the hope, however, that some compromise might be reached that would be a step in the direction I wished to go, I tried to define exactly what I wanted. My proposal to the members of the subsection read as follows:

---

*It should be pointed out that the word "euthanasia" is of Greek origin and means literally "a painless, happy death." This is the context in which the Euthanasia Educational Council uses the term. The interpretation of euthanasia as mercy killing is, however, widespread, and probably contributes to the controversy and confusion over this whole issue [Editor].

Since medical science has been able to prolong life far beyond its normal span by artificial means, but has *not* been able to stop the gradual deterioration of the body and the physical pain and mental anguish concomitant with terminal old age, termination of these artificial means for the prolongation of life shall no longer be termed "murder" or "suicide," but "death by natural causes"; that faced with the indignity of deterioration, dependence, physical pain and/or mental anguish, the patient has the *right* to ask that drugs be mercifully administered to hasten the moment of death; and that in case the patient no longer retains consciousness to express verbally the final decision but has recorded in writing his desire for death with dignity, it shall be mandatory that this request be honored and that lethal drugs be administered in accordance with his expressed desire.

This proposal was voted down in the subsection, as I expect it would have been even if the subsection had not been on spiritual well-being and been composed largely of clergy and representatives of religious institutions. The only action acceptable to the group was recognition of the individual's right to die with dignity. One delegate wanted to know how I could suggest hastening death when the Declaration of Independence guaranteed life, liberty, and the pursuit of happiness but made no mention of death. When I suggested that death is a part of life and that the individual's life is his own, he pointed to the legal injunction against suicide.*

---

*Some states suggest that individual liberty to control one's self and one's life does extend even to the liberty to end one's life. A 1954 decision frequently cited reads: "In those states where attempted suicide has been made lawful by statute (or the lack of one), the refusal of necessary medical aid (to one's self), whether equal to or less than attempted suicide, must be conceded to be lawful" [1].

Who Has the Right to Decide?

To the proposal that the patient should have the right under certain circumstances to ask that lethal drugs be administered to hasten the moment of death, it has been objected that no doctor would ever subscribe to this. The vital question is: Who has the veto power over prolongation of life? If you say the patient has that right, "provided his condition is hopeless and there is no chance of betterment," you give the veto to the doctor who decides whether there is a chance or not. This is just what I want to avoid, and I insist that it must be avoided. Of course such a right should not be exercised by the patient without careful consultation with the physician. After that the patient should have the right to decide for himself.

I recognize that the decision to cease prolonging life raises all kinds of difficulties. A person is despondent and says he wants to die. A young person has cancer, but there is the possibility, very remote perhaps, of a cure. Even in the aged (the aging are never called "aged" except in the last extremity) there is a hope for betterment.

At the Twenty-Fourth Annual Conference on Aging (1971) conducted by the University of Michigan and Wayne State University Institute of Gerontology [4], I debated with a physician, the director of a home for retired persons, on the right to die with dignity. I argued on the theoretical level that a patient should have the right to put an end to a long, painful, terminal illness. He cited case after case in which the patient had wished to die; close friends and relatives had thought it best; but he, my opponent, had insisted on heroic measures and had been able to restore the patient to at least partial health for a limited period of time. His contention was that you never reach the point at which your condition is completely hopeless until you are dead.

In the general discussion that followed I asked him if, in looking back, he found he had always been right in his judgment. There was a long pause, and then he admitted that sometimes things had not turned out exactly as he had hoped. In other words, as I interpret it, sometimes a patient had been kept alive for some period uselessly; but, the argument is, surely it is better to have ten suffer and one regain health or partial health than to have all die including the one who might have been restored.

The law of diminishing returns applies here. For example, an aged woman, who had always smoked heavily, suffered in the hospital from recurring attacks of pneumonia. During each attack she was given penicillin and recovered but successively became weaker, had shorter periods of consciousness, and was less able to regain control of herself. Finally her eldest son, a doctor, requested the physician in charge of the case not to give penicillin next time she had pneumonia, and she then died. Pneumonia used to be called the friend of the aged because the attack was sudden, fever quickly brought unconsciousness, and the end was swift. What was meant was that *death* was the friend of the aged and pneumonia was the easy path. Now penicillin has taken that path away.

I don't think I reveal any secret when I say that doctors often quietly take away heroic measures and artificial means of prolonging life when the case is hopeless and the end is obviously near, particularly if the patient is in great pain.

Their jurisdiction for this is, I believe, that the situation is such that the best interest and welfare of the patient are no longer compatible with preserving his life at all costs.

The question here is whether the responsibility for this decision can be transferred to the patient. When the choice is whether or not to perform an operation, the patient is given the decision. He may be told in the case of an infection that amputation would save his life but cost his arm or his leg; without an operation his life is in danger. *He* decides whether he is willing to take the risk. The Christian Scientist can refuse blood transfusions and other forms of treatments on the basis of religious conviction. It is a long step to allow the patient to decide when artificial means of prolonging life should be terminated; a still longer step to allow him the right to ask for lethal drugs at his own discretion.

Against such permission a formidable array of authorities is lined up, the most forbidding of whom is the doctor, because he has charge of the case and as such has the final say. All the *Living Will* can do is address each interested party in turn and beg each to respect the wish expressed in writing, namely that the person be allowed to die with dignity and a minimum amount of pain. The message is addressed first and appropriately to the family; and the family will be more difficult to convince even than the doctor, if the members are deeply attached to the patient.

Physicians give a number of reasons for not going along with a patient's decision to be allowed to die: medical practice and the honored precept of Hippocrates to preserve life, the legal aspects, and finally the family and friends who may veto all efforts at giving up the suffering patient.

The Tenets of Medical Practice

The details of medical practice and procedure differ somewhat from hospital to hospital. The Hippocratic oath, however, has been recognized as the basis of medical practice since the lifetime of Hippocrates or shortly thereafter (400 B.C.). In taking the Hippocratic oath the physician swears "to exercise his art solely for the cure of his patients"; and he swears by "whatever he holds most sacred," so that his oath is closely tied to whatever religion or deity he may support. Perhaps it is well to review the whole oath to see exactly what it demands of the honorable physician.

You do solemnly swear, each man by whatever he holds most sacred, that you will be loyal to the profession of medicine and just and generous to its members; that you will lead your lives and practice your art in uprightness and honor; that into whatsoever house you shall enter, it shall be for the good of the sick to the utmost of your power, you holding yourselves far aloof from wrong, from corruption, from the tempting of others to vice; that you will exercise your art solely for the cure of your patients and will give no drug, perform no operation, for a criminal purpose, even if solicited, far less suggest it; that whatsoever you shall see or hear of the lives of men which is not fitting to be spoken, you will keep inviolably secret. These things do you swear. Let each man bow the head in sign of acquiescence. And now, if you will be true to this, your oath, may prosperity and good repute be ever yours; the opposite, if you shall prove yourselves forsworn.

The ancient Greek, when ill, slept in the temple of Asklepius, and the god in a dream indicated the appropriate prescription for a cure. The physician-priest interpreted the dream, ministered to the suffering person's needs, and accomplished the cure. When the patient left the precinct, it was with the conviction (psychologically a very strong asset) that the god himself had recommended the appropriate treatment and would support the cure. Hippocrates writes as physician-priest but records only the symptoms observed and the cures employed.

Modern and ancient practices of medicine, of course, differ enormously. Ideas about the care and cure of many diseases have changed, and we have at our disposal a far greater number of cures, and an ability to prolong the life even of a person with an incurable disease far longer than was true in the days of Hippocrates. Furthermore one might argue that Greek and Roman society had a conception of the right to die with dignity. Suicide was accepted as a solution for a person disgraced or overcome with grief. It is possible also to point to the oath itself and say that, in the case of a patient tortured with disease or mental deterioration and with no reasonable hope of betterment, termination of life is "for the good of the sick," particularly if the patient desires it.

Too often, physicians seem committed to a philosophy of "cure" only, forgetting that "care" is an integral part of their role, and that when cure is no longer possible, the goal of treatment then becomes care and comfort until death ensues. Nowhere does the oath say that an incurably ill person must be kept alive indefinitely.

Influence of Religious Beliefs
Religious precepts are always cited as strong arguments in any discussion of the right to die. As part of a revealed

religion the principles of the Christian faith, for example, were expressed almost 2000 years ago and written down well over 1500 years ago. The precepts as contained in the Bible are open to interpretation, and there has been and still is a good deal of difference of opinion. Interpretations have changed, and I think one may foresee more changes in the future. On the other hand, among the convictions central to the Christian tradition, the prohibitions against murder and suicide seem unmistakable as evidenced, for example, by the Old Testament commandment, "Thou shalt not kill," which is as strong and valid an injunction today as it ever was.

Our views of death and dying are necessarily affected by our religious convictions and particularly by our conception of an afterlife. Even in ideas about afterlife, however, the precepts of a revealed religion can and do change through interpretation. The relationship between the physical body and the spirit is perhaps only indirectly concerned with the termination of life, but burial practice is very conservative in almost every religion and a change in practice is particularly slow. Through the centuries religions have upheld the sanctity of the body. Traditionally the dead body has been treated with respect, and preparations for burial, as well as the burial practices themselves, have been ritualized. Moreover, burial sites generally are looked upon as inviolable, and even today the grave that is interfered with in any way is said to be desecrated, a word which clearly describes the distaste with which such actions are perceived. The inviolability of the burial site seems to be tied more to the idea of the spirit and afterlife than to the corporate body itself.

An example of the sacredness of burial customs is the first settlement of New Haven, Connecticut, which was laid out in nine squares in accordance with the plan described in the Book of Revelations. Nine squares make a pattern with one square, the modern New Haven Green, in the center. Here was placed the cemetery (and later the churches), so that when the Day of Judgment dawned and the graves opened every good citizen of New Haven would be right there in the center of town and no one would be overlooked because his grave happened to be lost in the wilderness of early Connecticut.

It is doubtful that many people in the United States believe any more that the actual bones buried are going to rise again or that anyone not buried in a municipal center will be overlooked on the Day of Judgment. In fact, it is interesting to see how far the practice of cremation has penetrated our society. In Australia cremation is the usual custom, and a recent report from California stated that the high price of burial and cemetery lots was increasing the popularity of cremation and scattering of the ashes over the ocean.

Religious change, nonetheless, is notoriously slow. At the White House Conference the consensus of opinion among the delegates in the section Spiritual Well-Being of the Aging [5] was that the prolongation of life by artificial means was quite clearly in accordance with the will of God, but that hastening the moment of death even by the termination of artificial means for prolonging life was clearly in opposition to the divine decree. In the same Washington conference, however, of those committees devoted to special aspects of society and the needs of the aging, the Youth and Age Section proposed:

> Whereas young and old are one; and both deserve dignity and respect; and together are concerned with quality of life in the future as well as in the present; recognizing the urgency of the situation, we propose the following: That all persons, particularly the aging, be given the legal right to choose to die naturally and in dignity, avoiding prolonged illness, pain, confinement and degradation.

Another straw in the wind is the statement of Pope Paul in 1970. Although supporting the view that euthanasia without the patient's consent was murder and with his consent suicide, Pope Paul added that while doctors must fight death with all their resources, they were not obliged to use all the survival techniques known to science. Prolongation of life in some cases, he said, could be useless torture.

Could not the American belief in freedom of religion and the right of an individual to choose and follow his own beliefs be extended to include an individual's right to die with dignity — without that right being dependent on the beliefs of the physician, family, or any members of society? At the present time artificial means for prolonging life are in short supply: hospitals are crowded, the number of nurses is limited, respirators are few. If one patient gave up his demand for the respirator, intravenous feeding, and other heroic means for preserving life, then these facilities would be available for another. If, then, someone who interprets God's will in terms that do not stress the preservation of life at all costs, if *such a person* exercises his right to hasten the moment of death, and as a result a person with a more orthodox view is able to use these miracle means of preserving life, then surely he should be allowed to die in peace.

I have not mentioned expense, because human life cannot be measured in terms of money. With the short supply of hospital space and staff, however, comes the increased cost of hospitalization as one more worry for the conscientious patient. One may say, at least, that mental anguish caused by mounting expenses and particularly expenses not justified in terms of life expectancy, augmented by continued and increasing physical pain, adds one more cogent argument for granting the patient the right to die with dignity and a minimum amount of pain.

Legal Constraints

I place lawyers on the conservative side of this question because back of the lawyers is the law with a capital L, a law that changes very slowly, at least compared with the rate of modern developments in science and medical techniques. Behind the law are the fundamental principles embodied in the Constitution and the Declaration of Independence. It is the Declaration of Independence that asserts the inalienable rights of life, liberty, and the pursuit of happiness. Some believe that since it says nothing about death, there is no right to die.

A very nice point is raised by the "independence" argument. The Declaration asserts the right to the pursuit of happiness; it does not guarantee happiness, just the right to pursue it. In our declaring the right to die with dignity, what we are asking is the right to escape hopeless pain,

helpless indignity, and mental deterioration. I believe em-
phatically that "pursuit of happiness" in its broader sense
includes, as an essential element, the attempt to escape
from hopeless pain.

In a recent legal case in Florida [2], a woman of seventy-two
was hospitalized with a fatal form of blood disease. To keep
her alive surgical incisions had to be made in her veins for
almost continual blood transfusions, and she begged her
doctor to be allowed to die. The doctor took the case to
court to avoid the charge of aiding and abetting suicide on
the one hand or treating a patient against her will on the
other. The judge's decision stated that "a person has the
right not to suffer pain. A person has the right to live or
die in dignity." He ruled therefore that a patient could not
be forced to accept any treatment that was painful. The
transfusions were stopped, and a day later the patient died.
(For legal decisions involving similar cases see "Power of
the Courts" [3].)

So the law, like the church, does move; and a firm corner-
stone of our nation, the Declaration of Independence, may
be interpreted in more than one way.

I think the phrase *when life draws to a close* expresses
an essential part, at least for the time being, of the request
for the right to die with dignity. This avoids the question
of the despondent person, the disgraced, the disfigured, the
imbecile. The younger person stricken by an incurable disease and in increasing pain also deserves the right to hasten
death, but the weight of the argument becomes proportion-
ately greater the closer a person is to reaching the normal
expectancy of life. If anyone deserves such a right, it is the

aged first. Once the right has been granted to them, one may consider other cases.

The phrase *when life draws to a close* also raises questions: How do we know when life draws to a close? How do we know when there is no chance of betterment? The normal span of life is recognized and so is the fact of normal, gradual deterioration, physical and mental. Let us say, then, that we are concerned first with the aged patient afflicted with a painful incurable disease. Even so the doctor has an extremely difficult decision to make and the nurse a difficult role to undertake, because the instinct to live is strong and hope still flickers as long as life exists. The patient may have the *right* to die with dignity; but the decision should be made only after careful consultation with the doctor; and the advice to die, even consent to the decision to die, is not easy to give.

A Good Death

I do not want to minimize the difficulties for the patient himself. It would be easier were he to lapse into a coma and be allowed by the doctor to die in accord with his wish. But let us say that such is not his fate. Instead he finds himself in the hospital, growing weaker, and in constant pain. He knows the end cannot be far away, and he tells the nurse that he has consulted with the doctor and they are agreed it would be best for him to bring his hopeless pain to an end. It will not do at this point for the doctor to say that lethal drugs will be administered when he is asleep or may be concealed in food or medicine. The patient would become instinctively afraid of both doctor and nurse and suspicious of their every move.

I imagine the doctor coming in after the consultation has been concluded and the decision made, and saying quietly:

"Those pills you requested are on the table beside you, with a glass of water."

"Thank you, doctor."

"Is there anything else?"

"No, thank you, doctor."

"Good night, then."

"Good night." The patient is left alone with the lethal pills and the glass of water, and in the semi-darkness he has only one thought:

"I wish I were dead!"

The road to death is dreary, sad, and lonely, and the final decision most difficult, no matter how much one has steeled himself to it beforehand. Neither doctor nor nurse should urge or encourage the patient to take the final step. The patient makes the final decision. When he determines to exercise his right to die with dignity, the doctor administers the drugs or directs the patient in taking the final dose.

A Personal Plea for a Good Death

If I were to formulate my White House Conference proposals again, I should spell them out more explicitly and suggest that the Declaration of Independence of the United States includes the right to avoid pain and indignity in its provision of the right to the pursuit of happiness. I would ask, then, the right to escape from pain and indignity, mental anguish, and cerebral deterioration, when life draws to a close. There remains a vast gap between theory and practice. All might agree in principle that at some point the termination of exhausting life in a dying patient is a benefit rather than a calamity. Finding that point in practice is far from easy, but it should be tried.

My father died suddenly of a heart attack when he was seventy-five; his twin brother, a doctor, lived to be ninety but became both deaf and blind. His devoted wife cared for him night and day. I do not know whether he remained eager to live and she remained eager to keep him alive. All I know is that, faced with permanent loss of sight and sound, I want the right to hasten the moment of death if, at that time, I choose to exercise it. Suppose that to my deafness and blindness pain is added, necessitating a serious abdominal operation. I refuse the operation and look for relief in death; but I don't die, and the pain increases. Then my mind begins to give way. At what point am I justified in saying, "I have had enough," and why should I not legally have the right to act accordingly and to call upon doctor and nurse to assist?

An old and good friend of mine was kept alive at seventy-nine by heroic means and with only occasional intervals of consciousness. The doctor came to his wife and asked whether her husband should be kept alive any longer. She asked if there were any chance of betterment. The answer was no. "Let him go, then," she said and he died.

I do not want such agonizing questions put to either my son or my daughter. I want the right to die with dignity and a minimum amount of pain and the right to hasten the moment of death whether that right is expressed orally or in a written statement previously prepared.

I appeal to you nurses, who are acquainted with the

problem at first hand and who are not lawyers, doctors, pastors, nor members of a particular patient's family; I appeal to you as competent, impartial, and understanding judges, and through you to the families of patients and beyond them to the public at large. We need a change in public sentiment so that the individual, whether or not he intends himself to use the right to die, will recognize that the right to die with dignity is good; that the proper exercise of it is commendable; and that the person who does hasten the moment of death under appropriate circumstances is not only sensible and wise but a benefactor to himself, his family, and his community.

The nurse is not primarily concerned with the problem of the patient's right nor the doctor's decision. The nurse sees the end approaching and is in a position to appreciate the suffering of the patient better even than relative, friend, or doctor. What the patient hopes for at this critical period is first understanding, then sympathy — not commiseration — and finally help in finding the strength to face the end steadfastly. There is fear and dread almost invariably, but mingled with them the clear, calm assurance that death comes inevitably to all.

I might compare life to a hurdle race. We go through grammar school and then college or specialized training. We have the challenge of making good at our chosen job or profession. If we are married, there are the joys and problems of every marriage; and with children we go through the successive steps again by proxy. At the end of the race there is the tapering off of retirement, when professional duties and the press of business have slackened their grip. There is, however, still the slowdown, the last lap, the restful twilight of leisure. We are satisfied with the race, we are proud of our accomplishments, and we hope for a quiet, peaceful, pleasant old age. We pray that we may end with dignity and courage.

Nature brings to an end every mortal life and prepares our way to the grave by gradually diminishing our strength, both mental and physical. The helplessness at the beginning of life cannot be avoided, but there is no reason why we could not and should not avoid utter and impotent helplessness at the end. After an active and happy life, I do not wish to have the end cribbed and confined and protracted with dreary hours and hopeless days. Surely one has the right to put an end to that state, destitute of strength and sensibility, which we all pray we may never reach.

Death is inevitable. Look forward for a moment to the last critical phase in your own lives, although the end may not seem credible now. Then consider who should have the right of choice.

"Never send to know for whom the bell tolls," as John Donne wrote, "it tolls for thee."

References

1. Cawley, C. C. Criminal liability in faith healing. *Minn. Law Rev.* 39:48, 1954.
2. Dilemma in Dying. *Time* 19 July 1971, p. 44.
3. Di Stasi, L. C., Jr., Power of Courts or Other Public Agencies to Order Compulsory Medical Care for Adult. In *Amer. Law Rep.* Ser. 3, vol. 9, pp. 1391–1398.
4. Twenty-Fourth Annual Conference on Aging, Institute of Gerontology, The University of Michigan and Wayne State University, Ann Arbor, Mich., June 1971.

5. White House Conference on Aging, Toward a National Policy on Aging. Vol. II, Bethesda, Md.: U.S. Government Printing Office, 1971, p. 245.

Bibliography

Fletcher, J. Ethics and euthanasia. *Am. J. Nurs.* 73:670, 1973.

Hendin, D. *Death as a Fact of Life.* New York: Norton, 1973.

Kass, L. R. Death as an event: A commentary on Robert Morison. *Science* 173:698, 1971.

Krant, M. J. *Dying and Dignity.* Springfield, Ill.: Thomas, 1975.

Maguire, D. C. *Death by Choice.* Garden City, N.Y.: Doubleday, 1974.

Mannes, M. *Last Rights.* New York: Morrow, 1974.

Morison, R. S. Death, process or event? *Science* 173:694, 1971.

Morison, R. S. The last poem: The dignity of the inevitable and necessary. *Hastings Cent. Stud.* 2:63, 1974.

Ramsey, P. *The Patient as Person.* New Haven, Conn.: Yale University Press, 1970.

Ramsey, P. The indignity of "death with dignity." *Hastings Cent. Stud.* 2:47, 1974.

Russell, O. R. *Freedom to Die.* New York: Behavioral Publications, 1975.

Schoenberg, B., et al. *Psychological Aspects of Terminal Care.* New York: Columbia University Press, 1972.

Weber, L. J. Ethics and euthanasia: Another view. *Am. J. Nurs.* 73:1228, 1973.

Williams, R. H. *To Live and To Die.* New York: Springer, 1974.

5. COPING WITH DEATH IN ACUTE CARE UNITS

Rita E. Caughill

Acute-care units in a hospital differ in many important ways from general patient care units. They are geared to intensive medical and nursing care of acutely ill patients; they are equipped with an array of complex, life-sustaining machinery; and they are staffed by personnel who are usually specially trained and highly skilled in delivering the care required by their very ill patients.

In these days of ever-increasing specialization a particular hospital may have several acute care units of equal importance. The three units found in most urban hospitals today and quite often in smaller rural areas as well are the cardiac care unit, the intensive care unit, and the emergency department. The threat of death in these acute care settings increases tension to a remarkable degree. Of all the hospital population, patients in these areas have the highest potential for death while still retaining "salvageability." It is precisely because the staff in these units are geared to the defeat of death and the salvaging of human life that the tensions exist. These nurses and physicians see themselves as "cure agents" with their ultimate goal the restoration of health or at least some degree of health. Obviously the staff cannot always win the battle. When death intervenes, special problems are created that may not be clearly defined or recognized by staff, much less dealt with effectively. These death-related problems will be examined here in relation to the patient, the family, and the nurse in turn.

The Patient
The Emergency Patient
In the emergency department death usually is a sudden, catastrophic event caused by an outside force. Whether

that causative force is a traumatic accident or a coronary occlusion, it is sudden, unexpected, and overwhelming. Saving lives is the primary function of this unit, and the physical needs of the patient may be so urgent and demanding that there is little time to think about his emotional needs.

Yet the patient who is admitted in critical condition may be well aware of the seriousness of his situation and in desperate need of some kind of meaningful communication. If he is unconscious or semiconscious, this makes it easier for everyone in terms of interacting with him. He may be in a state of physical and emotional shock and not really aware of what is happening to him. If, however, he is conscious but seems confused, he should be oriented to his situation calmly and in simple language that he can readily understand. As emergency nurse, you can do this without lengthy explanations or false reassurances; your tone of voice and manner of speaking should provide the assurance that you care about him and will try to help him. Empty phrases such as "You'll be OK, don't worry" should be avoided. They may make *you* feel better, but they do nothing for the anxious patient.

The patient who is aware and concerned about his prognosis presents a different kind of problem. He may not say anything, only plead with his eyes for some answer, for reassurance. Even if he asks directly, "Am I going to die?" he may not really want the answer to that question. What he does want to know for certain is, first, that he is getting the best possible care and, then, that he is not going to be left alone. One of the greatest fears of a dying person

— or a person who suspects he may be dying — is the fear
of dying alone. Stay with him, and if you have to leave the
room, see that someone else remains there with him. More
than just being there, share yourself, meet his eyes, smile,
touch him, hold his hand, make him feel that you care about
him, not just his I.V.s or the myriad other gadgets that one
tends to become absorbed in to avoid that human contact
that means so much to the dying patient.

It is unfair to try to fool the patient who suspects he
will die; yet if he asks, "Am I dying?" it would be unwise
to answer "yes," as it might well destroy his will to fight
for life, often a critical factor in his survival. You might
reply that while his condition is serious and it is possible
that he could die, all of you are doing everything you can to
prevent it, and you need to have him fight, too. The
emergency patient is potentially salvageable, and it is important to maintain his hope and his will to live as a necessary
adjunct to the efforts to save him.

Kübler-Ross [12] maintains that a patient should never
be told that he is dying. Only when the patient himself
offers the information that he is fatally ill does she advise
talking openly to him about his dying. In the emergency
department, of course, patients are less likely to *tell* you
they are dying than to ask you, and their questions may be
prompted by fear, pain, suspicion, or by self-conviction
when they get no sensible response to their anxious queries.
You must try to assess what is behind the patient's questions, and of course your knowledge of what is actually
happening to him pathologically will also influence your
reply. It is essential to be very alert and sensitive to each

individual as you assess his need. Is he aware of what is happening to him? How much does he want to know? How much is he able to hear? Be honest in your reply, yet keep in mind that the whole truth may destroy him.

An important source of help and comfort for many patients is spiritual support. The Catholic patient who is in danger of death should always have a priest called. Patients of other faiths may or may not wish to have a clergyman attend them, but they should be given the choice. An appropriate time to suggest this might be when the patient is expressing concern about his possible death. If the patient does not verbalize such fears, the nurse must decide when to offer him this option. Some nurses hesitate to suggest a clergyman when the patient does not mention one, fearing that the suggestion will alarm the patient and thus do more harm than good. It is largely a question of weighing advantages against disadvantages. It seems unfair to deprive a patient of the comfort and strength he could derive from spiritual support simply because he is unable or reluctant to ask for it himself. The patient of opposite convictions, who has no interest in religious aid, may be alerted to his precarious status if this is offered to him, but he can then be reassured in keeping with his emotional response.

While religion may or may not be important to your patient, you cannot know this unless he tells you. If the patient does have strong religious convictions, these become far more important to him when his life is in danger, and if the patient dies, it will be a source of comfort to the family to know that spiritual guidance and support were provided.

The Patient in Acute Care Areas
In the intensive care unit and the coronary care unit the
acutely ill patient is a challenge to the whole team, and
death becomes an adversary that is fought with a high
degree of energy and skill. Unlike the emergency department, where the staff has little opportunity to get to know
a patient as a person, these units foster a close relationship
between patient and nurse. They are relatively small and
have a much lower patient-to-staff ratio than is found in the
average patient care areas of the hospital. As the patients
are there because they need almost continuous nursing
care, nurses are at the bedside much of the time. While the
turnover in patient population may be fairly rapid, many
patients remain there for days or weeks, and the longer they
are there, the harder it is for staff to cope if death is the
eventual outcome. The feelings of the nurse depend, of
course, on the closeness of the relationship she or he has
had with the patient.

In the coronary care unit (CCU) patients are usually alert
and oriented but dependent on the nurse for all aspects of
care, which results in closer relationships than are often
possible in the intensive care unit (ICU), where a hectic
pace is more constant. Patients generally may appear to be
in less critical condition, but this can change suddenly and
dramatically with an erratic ECG pattern or a cardiac arrest.

Patients in acute care units need realistic support at all
times. It is often difficult to determine, however, what is
realistic. Staff exert herculean efforts to save lives, and
they must believe it is possible to preserve the patient's life
in order to make the effort. Patients may already see their

situation as precarious, and no one wants to frighten them further by admitting the possibility that they could die. Still it must be remembered that the patient is the one person most affected by his own death! He deserves to know that it is possible, if in fact he really wants to know. On the other hand the patient whose prognosis is good deserves to know that as well. Too often staff unwittingly allow patients to lie in limbo, having no clear idea of their probable fate. It cannot be assumed that a patient is not thinking about death and fearful of it simply because he expresses no concern or even denies concern.

Two recent studies of fear of personal death [6, 7] found that even when individuals consciously denied fear of death, they were in fact quite fearful at the unconscious level. One of the studies focused specifically on patients who were dying from cancer or heart disease. This study reported that "patients close to impending death are markedly more afraid of death on an unconscious level than healthy individuals. This reality must be appreciated despite surface indications of a lack of manifest conscious fear" [7]. Needless to say, this kind of repressed anxiety can have serious consequences for the critically ill patient.

Cassem and Hackett [3, 9] further demonstrated the significance of denial as a defense mechanism used by patients with acute cardiac conditions. In a study of 100 patients hospitalized in a coronary care unit these investigators found that all but four claimed to have experienced little or no fear at any time during their hospitalization. Of this same group eleven witnessed a fatal cardiac arrest but managed to rationalize the death in various ways, with

no admission that the same thing could happen to them.
Furthermore patients who themselves survived cardiac
arrest have been found [4, 5, 9, 17] to use various defense
mechanisms to control their anxiety, the most common
being denial.

If denial is the coping mechanism the patient most often
uses in dealing with his situation, it is important for staff
to handle it appropriately. Hackett et al. [9] differentiate between *major deniers* and *partial deniers,* the
former being those who unequivocally deny having any
fear at all and the latter those who admit some fear or
anxiety at least some of the time during their stay in the
CCU. These investigators feel that the partial deniers may
want reassurance but are unable to communicate their
need. Nurses would do well, then, to begin with basic kinds
of reassurance, explaining to the patient every treatment
involved in his care and every aspect of the environment
that might appear strange, threatening, or foreboding.
Encouragement should be given in as specific terms as
possible. It is concrete and positive reassurance to say,
"Your pulse is slower and stronger today. That's a good
sign." By contrast a vague and airy comment like "You're
getting along fine" leaves room for much interpretation.
The patient who lies there and thinks about it may ultimately perceive it as totally false reassurance, and it will
only increase his anxiety. Overdoing encouragement and
reassurance can have the same negative effect; the patient
may interpret it as an attempt to conceal your own anxiety
about him: "She's trying so hard to reassure me, I must
be in really bad shape."

Sedation is useful in relieving fear and anxiety and may be indicated even in the major denier who does not appear to need it. Since it is difficult to know when a patient is truly and completely denying the serious nature of his illness, this patient should be given the same positive kinds of feedback as the one whose fear is more evident.

The patient who is able to talk should be encouraged to express his concerns. The patient who is not able to talk but who is conscious or semiconscious should be assured by the nurse that she is aware of his concerns and then given *realistic* assurance concerning his progress and prognosis. Ignoring the fact that he has anxieties fails to meet his most basic needs.

The Family

In all the acute care areas the family seems to be an unwelcome and neglected element. Families are usually viewed by the staff as a problem or even as a downright nuisance. Nurses complain about the repeated questions of anxious relatives, frequent telephone calls of inquiry, and similar demands on their time.

As a general rule families are allowed visiting privileges for only five minutes out of each hour, a meager allotment indeed when a loved member of the family is critically ill and possibly dying. Yet to allow them free access to a room that is already overcrowded with equipment and personnel would be unrealistic. Few families expect preferential treatment. The concept of acute care units with their limited visiting privileges is by now well known to the public and accepted at least in theory. Abiding by those rules can be nerve-wracking for an emotionally involved person, however, and staff should make every effort to be sensitive to the family's feelings. Often a warm smile and a sincere word of regret about the necessity for such rules will appease an anxious relative.

If there is a waiting room where families of critically ill patients can spend time, they are often very supportive of each other. The opportunity to share common problems and compare case histories gives all of them the chance to talk out some of their concerns and can be very therapeutic. If the nurse can take time occasionally to share information with the family and be supportive in doing so, the family's needs will be met at least partially. Nonverbal communication to the family may be much more meaningful than verbal, since there is often little new to tell them. Kindness and warmth really take no more time than restraint and formality.

Where efforts to include the family have been tried, results have been positive and rewarding. Baden [1] found, for example, that daily phone calls to the family to report on the CCU patient's status not only improved relationships between nurse and family but resulted in fewer incoming calls to the unit. Another important advantage of such a system is that the nurse controls the timing of the calls, thus avoiding interruptions of routine at awkward or busy times. It is worth keeping in mind, too, that people under stress may remember little of what is told them, so that while repeating the same information may be monotonous to the nurse, it usually is not perceived this way by the recipient.

Nurses in an acute care unit may feel torn between the time required for care of their patients and the time it would take to comfort an anxious spouse or family member. As one nurse stated, "No one recognizes the family as their responsibility. Much of what the nurse sees as intrusion and nagging stems from anxiety and ignorance of what is going on. Often this could be controlled with just a few words of reassurance." Families *are* an essential part of total patient care. The family's emotional tone is quickly transmitted to the patient and can have profound effects on his physical and psychological state.

Coping with the Family's Grief
In the event of patient death the crisis situation for the family is similar in all acute care units. In the emergency department, however, the grief reaction is likely to be more acute, because the death occurs so soon after the precipitating event and is almost totally unexpected. It is a true emergency situation for the survivors, and it is urgently important that staff give them all possible help as they face this crisis. The death has come as a terrible shock to them, and their reactions may be difficult for the staff to deal with. Especially if they become highly emotional and noisy or angry and unreasonable, the staff may well wish they would sign the necessary papers and leave, to do their grieving at home.

It will help to understand them and accept their behavior, even to comfort them more effectively, if one keeps in mind the symptoms and characteristics of the acute grief reaction. (See Chapter 2.) In the initial reaction of shock

and denial the person may not only cry out, "No, it can't
be true!" but also try to disavow the fact in other ways: by
throwing himself on the body, for example, as though this
will somehow restore life — or as though he believes that
life is still there. Cultural patterns determine to some extent
the amount of public crying and lamentation that people
will indulge in; some ethnic groups are very open in their
expressions of emotion, while others tend to be more re-
strained. At a time of acute grief, cultural practices are
extremely important and should never be discouraged,
criticized, or belittled in any way.

Regardless of race, ethnic background, *or sex,* crying is a
legitimate release in the presence of death. We not only
accept crying, we expect it; and we are not — or should not
be — shocked at the sight of a man's tears under these
circumstances.

The anger characteristic of the second stage of grieving
may be openly displayed by the survivors of sudden, unexpected death. It may be directed at the doctor, the nurse,
the hospital; someone, they feel, must have "botched the
job" and allowed the loved one to die. Staff should be
aware that this anger is rarely directed at them personally,
although it may appear to be; it is more a manifestation of
the individual's feelings of frustration and helplessness, of
an inability to *do* anything about it. Anger may be felt
toward another family member who somehow failed in his
obligation toward the deceased. Or it may be directed
against the individual himself, if he feels himself to be at
fault. Parents especially tend to feel guilt over the death
of a child and may berate themselves or each other or may

even injure themselves in an impulsive gesture of aggression or self-destruction. Guilt in fact is probably felt to some degree by all bereaved persons, as they search their minds for ways in which they may have failed the loved one, when it is now too late to make amends.

Notifying the Family of the Death

Who announces the death to the family? And how? If at all possible, it is helpful to give the family some advance warning that things are not going well, that death seems imminent and inevitable. This allows at least some brief time for the family to work through some of their feelings before the final blow, death, actually arrives. Families of patients who die a lingering death have time to go through a good deal of their grief work beforehand, so that when the patient finally dies, they may already be into the third, restorative stage of grieving. When death is sudden and unexpected, however, there is little or no time for preparatory grieving, and the shock is then much greater. If the nurse can report periodically how things are going, even if the news is progressively worse each time, this is far better than no reporting at all. Sudden death is a grim fact which must be accepted; avoiding the family or offering false hope is not helpful.

It is almost always better if the physician tells the family of the death. He or she is the person whom the relatives see as the primary authority. They have the opportunity to ask questions if they wish and to ask advice about immediate problems they may have. Even if the physician has never had any previous contact with the family, which is often the case, he can still establish a meaningful relationship with the survivors in a very short time. Many doctors defend the position that they should not have to become involved with the family after a death, maintaining that their responsibility is to the living and that when the patient dies, their responsibility ends. But the grieving relatives are living and urgently in need of support.

Nurses often feel that they are better equipped to inform families than physicians are, that their nurturing role enables them to show their concern and sympathy more effectively, and that they are more supportive of the grief-stricken kin. This may be true in many cases, and if the task does fall to a nurse who is comfortable in the role, the family surely benefits from her (or his) touch. Nevertheless it is still important that the family have contact with a physician who has been in attendance on the deceased person. If no physician is in evidence, they will be left to speculate as to whether a doctor was ever present, and the thought that their loved one might have been saved if a competent doctor had been available may torment them for all time. The physical presence of a physician with whom they can talk will reassure them that everything possible was done. The nurse can certainly accompany the physician if she wishes, can temper explanations if she feels that is necessary, and can stay with the family after the doctor leaves, to explain, amplify, and reinforce the information given them.

When the family is not present and must be summoned by telephone, the problem is somewhat different. Most professionals agree that if the death has been sudden and

completely unexpected, the family should not be notified
by phone. It is impossible for the staff member on one end
of the phone to know what the situation is on the other end.
Heart attacks have been precipitated and acts of self-injury
or even self-destruction have been attempted by distraught
survivors who were alone when the devastating news came.
Furthermore the harried relatives, in their haste to reach
the hospital, may themselves become the victims of an
automobile accident en route.

The all-important factor in phoning the family, if there
is no other immediate way to notify them, is to keep calm.
The nurse sets the stage for the way in which the family
reacts. If she can quietly convey the information that there
has been an accident and that they should come to the hospital as soon as they can, but with no urgency in her voice,
chances are that they will be able to avoid panic. They will
of course be alarmed and may immediately expect the
worst; but even if they ask if it is serious or if the patient is
dead, she can still avoid the whole truth without lying by
saying, perhaps, "He has been badly injured, but everything
possible is being done. There is no need for you to rush."
When they arrive and there is face-to-face contact, the
nurse again tries to control the situation by being very composed and calm in her approach. What has happened should
be explained clearly and in terms that they can understand,
emphasizing the quality of care that was given. Again, the
physician should speak with the family, even if it means
having to wait for their arrival.

It is always better if another member of the family, or
perhaps a close friend, is also present. They provide support

109

for each other, and grief that is shared is somehow easier to
bear. In any case the bereaved should not be left alone. If
it is the nurse who breaks the news to the family, and she
is *really* too busy to remain long with them (and not simply
looking for an excuse to escape from this uncomfortable
situation), some reasonable substitute must be found — a
chaplain or spiritual advisor, perhaps. Even an aide who is
a warm, concerned individual can fulfill this role with a
little training and a lot of support.

Viewing the Body
Should the family be allowed to see the body? Nurses often
feel that if there is severe mutilation, especially of the head
or face, it is too shocking a sight for the family to endure.
Difficult as it is, it is necessary and desirable if the family is
to face the death as a reality. Studies have shown that the
survivors who have the most difficulty resolving their grief
are those who never get to see the body, because of drown-
ing, an airplane crash, or other tragedy where the body was
never recovered.

After a hospital death then, the body should be cleansed,
cleared of tubes and other resuscitative devices, and made
as presentable as possible. At least some identifiable part
should be visible for the relatives, to confirm the loss. They
should be prepared ahead of time so that they will have
some idea what to expect, but they should always be given
this option. It is a form of reality orientation which the
numbed survivors need.

The following two instances illustrate this. One is the
case of a young woman who lost a very dear brother in an

automobile accident. His body was sent immediately across the country to the city where their parents had moved, and it was buried there. The sister never saw his body and has never seen his grave. Although many years have passed, she still resents her mother "taking Donny away from me." She feels he should have been buried where she is, but when asked if she has thought of going to visit his grave, she resists the idea and still irrationally blames her mother for the loss.

The father of another young woman died when she was about twelve years old, and his body was cremated. She had not even seen him while he was sick and hospitalized. His death is unreal to her, despite the fact that his ashes repose in an urn on the mantelpiece. The family plans to sprinkle the ashes from a plane (which was his wish), and then there will not even be ashes to confirm the fact of his death. This woman is in a state of partial denial of her father's death. She knows that he died, yet she has never had any proof of that fact and cannot really accept it.

Psychological Support
Many authorities recognize the pressing need in hospitals for some sort of psychological consultation service for bereaved families. Quint and others [14] see this as possibly a social worker's role, but they ask realistically, who would pay for the twenty-four-hour-a-day services of such a person? Is the public ready to assume the cost? While in some instances a chaplain may fill the role of comforter to the bereaved, it is important to realize that the mere fact of being a clergyman does not necessarily equip one to meet the

needs of people in the acute stages of grief. The chaplain,
too, needs special preparation, often not provided in religious training. Ryan [15] describes the role of a psychiatric
nurse as a regular member of the cardiac arrest team, assigned
to support the family through the crisis. The same function
could be performed by a regularly assigned nurse specially
trained for the role in communication skills and psychological principles. Kübler-Ross [12] suggests that volunteers
specially trained in grief work might be used effectively.
They would have the advantage of being uninvolved in the
effort to save the patient, which is so emotionally draining,
and could therefore devote all of their energies to comforting the family. Volunteers who have experienced grief in
their own lives are ideal workers with whom to start, and
they can readily be trained in basic psychological and communication techniques. They could be available on a
twenty-four-hour basis with no added cost to the hospital.

Another essential element, too often lacking in hospitals,
is a room where grieving relatives can be provided privacy.
Every area of the hospital should be able to provide such a
room, but certainly in high-risk areas it is indispensable.
To give the family shocking news in a corridor or in a waiting room filled with curious and perhaps anxious observers
is heartless and inexcusable. If no space is set aside for this
specific purpose, a nearby chapel, office, or any small empty
room might be used. Hospitals now being built or reno-
vated should include one or more such "crying rooms."

Survivors must be allowed, indeed encouraged, to express
their acute grief in whatever way it comes out. Whether it
is noisy or subdued, accept their tears or anger without

comment. Touch is extremely effective in conveying sympathy and concern — an arm around the shoulders, a handclasp. A simple offer of services: "Can I get you a glass of water?" "How about a cup of hot coffee?" "Can I phone your sister to come and be with you?" What you say is not so important as how you say it. What you do is not so important as that you be there.

Sociologist David Sudnow [16] studied practices surrounding death in a large county hospital in California. One of his observations that seemed particularly sad was this: "In none of the cases I have observed did the physician touch the relative or attempt to say anything while the relative was crying. No sympathy remarks or gestures of sorrow were offered during the earliest period following his announcement" of death [16, p. 141]. In this study, the "physicians" were almost always young residents. It is not professionally demeaning to say "I'm sorry" or even to shed a tear with the bereaved if one is so moved.

Sedating the grieving relatives is not always a good idea. Physicians and nurses have to be very honest in looking at their own actions and reactions, especially when following practices that "have always been done this way." Sedation does quiet the sobbing and appears to help people "get hold of themselves." It may, however, only serve to delay the grief reaction. It would be far better to allow the bereaved to cry and express their rage and frustration where there is a shoulder to cry on, where they can vent their anger without injuring themselves. It is difficult to help people who are irrational with hurt and anger; it is easier to send them home, get them "out of your hair." If you can be patient and understanding, perhaps agree that you would probably feel the same way if it happened to you, then they may be able to recover to the point where they can be sent home safely. But no individual should go alone. The survivor who is utterly alone in the world, with no relative, no friend, no minister, not even a neighbor who can stay with him, is a very real problem. Many people in acute states of anguish are suicidal for a time. It would be better to admit such a person overnight, in the care of nurses who are warm and compassionate, with the hope and expectation that he will be able to cope the next day. This is idealistic? Perhaps, but why should ideals always be brushed aside as impossible? Many things become possible when someone really believes they are important and necessary.

The Nurse

Nurses in acute care settings must act under enormous pressures. The fact that they must work hard, react promptly, and make important decisions on the spot adds to the tension but at the same time helps them maintain composure in critical situations. They see their role as a lifesaving one, primarily. Death is usually viewed negatively, as failure. Sometimes, when a close relationship has been formed between nurse and patient, it is a personal loss and a personal failure. When many deaths occur in a short span of time, the effect may constitute a disaster, and few nurses can handle their feelings without adequate support. Yet opportunities are seldom provided for staff to work through their feelings. Rarely does anyone think to reassure the nurse that she or he is indeed functioning at a high level and is not a failure in a given situation.

Cassem and Hackett [3] explored in detail the many sources of psychological stress for the CCU nurse. Some of their suggestions for amelioration of problems included increased communication with co-workers (sharing of mutual concerns) and availability of a physician or nurse clinician to share the enormous responsibilities they often are forced to face alone. In my experience, coping with crises alone has been the major source of stress and distress to CCU nurses. Theoretically, they say, physicians and supervisors are always available, but in fact they often do not arrive for several minutes after the need arises. By that time the nurse has already defibrillated the patient and taken on all the necessary responsibility herself. While nurses derive satisfaction from successful efforts of this kind, they are at the same time weighed down by the heavy burden of responsibility. Unsuccessful efforts can lead to demoralizing feelings of helplessness.

Involvement with the Patient
Many other factors contribute to the psychological stresses on nurses in acute care settings. When a patient is in the unit for any length of time, a growing social story [8] begins to unfold which makes him or her a unique person to the staff and adds to the poignancy they experience in caring for the patient. The more personal information about the patient that becomes known to the staff, concerning family background, occupation, personality, and so forth, the more clearly a person that patient becomes. Personal involvement of the staff grows as the social history grows. This can occur whether or not the patient is conscious and able to communicate with the staff.

A typical example is the story of Donny, a teenager who sustained serious internal injuries in an accident on his parents' farm. Despite their rural background both the boy and his parents adjusted very well to the busy environment of the intensive care unit and were always pleasant and appreciative of the doctors' and nurses' efforts. It did not occur to the staff for some time that this brave young man might not pull through. As his condition steadily worsened, they redoubled their efforts to save him. They admired his parents' strong religious faith and found themselves praying, too, for his recovery. They bent the rules regarding the five minutes each hour allowed for visiting, so that Donny's parents could remain with him for longer periods. The boy could not talk because of a tracheostomy, he could not write because of intravenous needles, yet he always had a smile to greet them and always cooperated with treatments. It was only after he had suffered two respiratory arrests and the doctor said his lung was too badly damaged to do anything more that the reality of the situation hit them.

"I knew I was going to cry," one nurse related. "I just couldn't accept the truth that Donny was going to die. The atmosphere of the whole unit was gloomy. I wasn't assigned to Donny the day he died. I tried to concentrate on my work, but I couldn't keep my mind off Donny. I just remember his parents sitting at his bedside, talking to him in a soothing way. They were so strong. If it hadn't been for them we all would have been emotional wrecks.... After Donny died and his parents had left, we all broke down and cried. It really drained me emotionally."

The social loss value of this young patient was very much a factor here. But the same intense emotional involvement can occur whenever the patient's developing story is interesting, unusual, or appealing for any reason. Staff then feel personally involved in the situation and may be deeply touched by it.

Many patients are warm and magnetic and involve the

staff in a deeper emotional attachment than ordinarily is developed. This was true in the following case.

An attractive, middle-aged woman was admitted to the emergency department with severe chest pain, which was subsequently determined to be a coronary occlusion. She remained in the emergency department for some three hours before a bed was available on a unit and in this time became much more comfortable. She was very friendly and likeable, and since the staff were not busy, they spent a lot of time with her. When she was finally transferred to a unit, they discussed her chances of recovery and all hoped she would get along well, "since she was such a lovely person." About an hour later a "code 5" was sounded. The emergency department staff sensed that it could be "their patient" and waited anxiously to find out. When they learned that it was indeed this gracious woman and that she had died, the staff was overcome with gloom. For the remainder of the shift, everyone went about his own duties in silence, deep in his own thoughts.

Nurses and physicians are exposed to other kinds of emotional trauma. Often they identify closely with the patient or with a member of the family. A woman who is the same age as the nurse, a child who is as young as her own child, an older man who reminds her of her father — these are the ones who bring the tragedy closer to the nurse's own life and heighten the impact of their deaths upon her.

Nurses' Need for Support

Sometimes it is the family members that upset the staff as much as the patient does. They may be excessively demanding, hysterical, and noisy in their lamentations. Possibly the hardest to tolerate is the family that accuses the staff of negligence or even of causing their loved one's death. Adding to the dilemma is the staff's difficulty in coping with their own feelings after a death. They are tired, frustrated, and drained by their unsuccessful efforts. What they really need is a chance to ventilate their own feelings, but instead they must maintain their composure and attempt to calm the family.

Members of the staff who have suffered a recent bereavement of their own may have great difficulty in coping with dying patients and their families. They need help in handling their own problems — an opportunity to discuss their own loss as well as the work experiences that have upset them.

Even though she is specially trained and highly competent, it seems unfair to expect the acute care nurse to carry on without adequate support from persons with greater knowledge and competence than hers. Too often she is taken for granted and treated as though she has no needs of her own. Nurses themselves may suppress their emotional needs on the assumption that these are luxuries they cannot afford. Patient care inevitably suffers, however, for the nurse cannot give support to others if she herself has no one to turn to for support.

Sharing feelings with peers can be a helpful release, but more than this seems necessary. Kornfeld [10] suggests regular conferences of the head nurse with her staff, and this certainly would be helpful if the meetings were used to share feelings at a gut level and to work through feelings of frustration and inadequacy. This is not always an easy thing to do, and any kind of successful resolution of problems requires a leader who is skilled in eliciting covert feelings, and then skilled in handling the results.

Kübler-Ross [13] suggests that every unit should have a "screaming room," a term she uses to describe a room set aside for staff, both medical and nursing, to use when the going gets tough, where they can relax, share their frustrations, get support from colleagues, and cry if they feel like it.

Benoliel [2] expresses the interesting theory that many nurses, as students, were first exposed to grief-provoking situations under circumstances which forced them to block expression of their grief, resulting in postponement of the grief reaction, an abnormal response. If nurses are indeed functioning with unresolved grief carried over from earlier experiences, this might well account for some of the inappropriate responses to death and grief that frequently are seen — notably maintaining social distance and a stiff professional demeanor. Some students are fortunate enough to receive adequate support in their early contacts with death and loss and are enabled to express their grief at the time. Benoliel postulates that these nurses are then able to be compassionate, supportive caregivers. But because of repeated exposure to death, loss, and grief throughout their professional practice, resolution of loss may never be complete for many practitioners.

Staff should be helped to understand that this kind of problem exists. They should be encouraged to look into their own backgrounds for experiences with dying patients that have been traumatic for them, and then helped to work through their feelings.

Summary and Conclusions

Medical and nursing care have achieved high levels of development, and professional caregivers have remarkable expertise in delivering complex care as long as they can expect the normal rewards of success (i.e., recovery). But when the outcome of their efforts is death, the feeling is one of failure and defeat. Nowhere is this attitude more apparent than in the acute care areas of the hospital, where dying is viewed with consternation and dismay, as something that should not be allowed to happen.

Staff need help, first, in recognizing that a problem exists, second, in learning to cope with the problem. Many nurses, despite repeated exposure to death, have never come to grips with their own feelings about it. If they are struggling with their own anxieties about death, they will find it difficult to help their patients cope with theirs.

It would seem that a great deal of concentrated effort is required to effect change and achieve the full potential for meaningful, supportive care. A few general suggestions follow, applicable to any of the acute care settings.

Staff need to become aware of their own feelings about death. A program for developing this awareness might be initiated by personnel in continuing education, by psychiatric nurses, or by consultants. Any number of films, film strips, audiotapes, books, and articles are available to facilitate the process.

Staff must be helped to see in realistic terms the extent of their own capabilities and the limitations of their care. In other words they need to recognize that death is inevitable and will occur in certain cases despite the best efforts of anyone and everyone.

While it is important to sympathize and empathize with patients and their families, it is equally important to be able to pull back and look at the situation objectively. Staff must know how to take one day at a time, and when they leave it, really leave it behind. They must learn to use time away from the hospital as therapy, in order to return refreshed and renewed.

It would seem worthwhile to look into the possibility of rotating nurses out of acute care areas at intervals. While such a policy rarely meets with approval from nurses, the long-term benefits are substantial with respect to renewed enthusiasm and rejuvenation. One hospital recently conducted an intensive two-week workshop for twenty-five members of its nursing staff selected from all over the hospital. The express purpose of the learning experience was to enable this group to function in any of the acute care areas should the need arise. This would seem an ideal and relatively simple way of providing relief personnel for one or two nurses at a time to rotate out of these highly stressful areas for whatever interval of time seems necessary. It could obviate much of the insensitivity to patients' needs which develops as an ego defense after prolonged periods of exposure to critically ill or dying patients.

As mentioned earlier, one should not overlook the potential of volunteers as support persons for the family. Volunteers should be carefully selected for this work, given sufficient training, and provided with support when they need it. In order to function effectively, they should be given a report on the patient and the family each time they come in, so that they are prepared for changes in the family's attitude and outlook.

Sociologists Glaser and Strauss [8] suggest that the staff of *every* hospital unit, but especially the high-risk areas, should sit down and examine closely the typical dying trajectory in their unit and the reaction patterns of various staff members when a death occurs: Who does what, who should do what, where the problems are, how they might be solved. Who is the strongest member of the team? The weakest? How can they help each other to improve not only the care but the emotional climate of the unit? They should all sit down together and get out their feelings and emotions, support each other, help each other. This means doctors, nurses, aides, orderlies, everyone who is a part of the unit's function. Every member of the staff needs to talk with the others as human beings, forgetting the hierarchy which for years has prevented physicians from sharing their feelings with nurses and has made nurses feel they must maintain an air of cool detachment as a part of their professionalism.

All hospital staff members experience grief, anger, shock, and frustration in their work. All need support. Staff generally are surprised at how much it helps to admit this openly and share their feelings with each other. In every group in which discussions of death and dying have been purposely initiated, the reaction expressed after only a few sessions is invariably, "I thought I was the only one who felt this way! I never knew other people had the same feelings I had." And everyone feels better just knowing that.

In addition to team conferences role play is a very useful tool in improving communication with the dying and the bereaved. Groups usually need assistance in getting this started but usually can be helped by the Continuing Education Department, if the hospital has one.

Initiating any of this activity is difficult, and first attempts will be painful and may appear futile. A particular situation may require psychiatric counseling or may benefit from pastoral counseling. Help is available if the staff is willing to look for it; ultimately their greatest strength will come from each other.

After a time, as staff members gain perspective into their feelings about death, they can look at ways of best helping dying patients and their families. It is only by working together in this way that they can come to grips with their own anxieties about death, integrate death into the process of living, and help those who truly need help at a time of great personal crisis.

References

1. Baden, C. Pointers coronary patients have given me for improving their care. *Consultant* 9:45, 1969.
2. Benoliel, J. Q. Anticipatory Grief in Physicians and Nurses. In Schoenberg, B., et al. (Eds.), *Anticipatory Grief.* New York: Columbia University Press, 1974.
3. Cassem, N. H., and Hackett, T. P. Sources of tension for the CCU nurse. *Am. J. Nurs.* 72:1426, 1972.
4. Cassem, N. H., et al. Reactions of coronary patients to the CCU nurse. *Am. J. Nurs.* 70:319, 1970.
5. Druss, R. G., and Kornfeld, D. S. Survivors of cardiac arrest. *J.A.M.A.* 201:291, 1967.
6. Feifel, H., and Branscomb, A. B. Who's afraid of death? *J. Abnorm. Psychol.* 81:282, 1973.
7. Feifel, H., et al. Death fear in dying heart and cancer patients. *J. Psychosom. Res.* 17:161, 1973.

8. Glaser, B. G., and Strauss, A. *Time for Dying.* Chicago: Aldine, 1968.
9. Hackett, T. P., et al. The coronary-care unit. *N. Engl. J. Med.* 279:1365, 1968.
10. Kornfeld, D. S., et al. Psychological hazards of the intensive care unit: Nursing care aspects. *Nurs. Clin. North Am.* 3:41, 1968.
11. Kübler-Ross, E. *On Death and Dying.* New York: Macmillan, 1969.
12. Kübler-Ross, E. *Lessons from the Dying Patient.* Flossmoor, Ill.: Ross Medical Association, 1973.
13. Kübler-Ross, E. Letter to a nurse about death and dying. *Nursing '73* 3:11, 1973.
14. Quint, J. C. (panelist). Symposium on managing the dying process. *Patient Care* 4:7, 1970.
15. Ryan, M. A. Helping the family cope with a cardiac arrest. *Nursing '74* 4:80, 1974.
16. Sudnow, D. *Passing On.* Englewood Cliffs, N.J.: Prentice-Hall, 1967.
17. White, R. L., and Liddon, S. C. Ten survivors of cardiac arrest. *Psychiatry Med.* 3:219, 1972.

6. THE DYING CHILD

Carol S. Green-Epner

Death is the unique and inevitable experience. It is a beginning according to the teachings of Catholicism; it is an end according to certain teachings of Judaism. It may be conceptualized as man's ultimate challenge — or his ultimate downfall.

The Death Taboo

In current American society considerable emphasis is placed on youth, health, power, and beauty. We are a future-oriented people who take pride in vim, vigor, and energy. Death, as the antithesis to these ideals, is a topic to be avoided. Death has been referred to as our most repressed reality. Its existence is ignored, isolated, or denied entirely. Gorer points out that mid-Victorian disgust and suppression of sexuality are now refocused on death [13]. Americans are loath to face death squarely, and our towering hospitals, medical centers, and research centers serve as a shining testimonial to our dedication to the prolongation of life.

This death taboo remains enforced within the realm of health professionals. We say that a person has "passed on," "passed away," "departed," "gone to sleep," "gone to heaven," or "expired," rather than that he has died. Feifel conducted a study in which he demonstrated that conversations about death were beneficial to the dying. Yet he received such strong opposition from the medical and nursing personnel that he was forced to conclude that this remained a very stressful area for them [9]. Kübler-Ross reported on her many encounters with physicians who were approached to determine if they would refer dying patients to her for counseling. She found that many of the physicians

125

were disbelieving, uncooperative, overprotective, and defensive [21]. Quint and Strauss found that nurses preferred clinical units where "the patients get well and go home" [37]. Kneisl reported on a study in which nurses hurried to answer the call lights of good-prognosis patients but were consistently slower in answering the call lights of poor-prognosis patients [20]. A patient's death may be viewed as a personal failure by many health professionals, as it frustrates their primary goal — cure. Whereas cure elicits social rewards, recognition, and reinforcement, death elicits frustration, anger, and guilt. The death of a patient has provoked feelings of negligence in many nurses.

The avoidance of death extends to the care of fatally ill children, also. In a study of twenty-six mothers whose children were dying, several questions were presented. Among them were: "Who was the most helpful person after you first learned that your child was not going to recover?" Only one mother mentioned a nurse. "Who was with your child when he died?" Again, only one mother mentioned a nurse [12].

Unfortunately the death taboo functions only to create an increasing number of problems for the dying child. A child's life style is characterized by a strong bond with his parents and an insatiable need for their continuous love, support, attention, and approval. He knows through his enculturation that to merit this affection he must exhibit behavior that is deemed appropriate (i.e., "good"). Illness may be viewed by the child as a consequence of inappropriate or "bad" behavior. Subsequent hospitalization and removal from his parents may be seen as the punishment for this wrongdoing. This places a serious strain on the child. When the constant loving attention of the parents is denied the child due to hospitalization, a period of grief ensues. Lindemann describes this grief as all-encompassing and pervasive. Sighing and other respiratory disturbances, lack of strength, diminished appetite, feelings of guilt, irritability, and loss of sociability are but a few of the symptoms [23]. Bowlby [4] discusses the separation anxiety the child will experience as comprising three phases: (1) protest, (2) despair, and (3) detachment. The child is frightened, lonely, anxious, and upset and may exhibit withdrawn, hostile, or regressed behavior.

The pronouncement of a terminal diagnosis upon the child causes the parents to retreat behind the death taboo with fervor. The parents present the child with a façade of forced cheerfulness and evasiveness. They make plans for his recovery and his return home. Unexpected gifts appear, especially those that the child has long desired but has been denied due to excessive cost or inaccessibility. The parents become more permissive and allow the child to skip naptime, extend bedtime, or omit a bothersome procedure. They become easily tearful, quickly leave the room, and then return bright, gay, and in high spirits. They avoid serious discussions of any kind and maintain superficial, lighthearted conversations. Through their actions and words the parents firmly and continuously deny to the child that anything is wrong.

The parents contend that they are protecting the child by keeping the truth from him. They attempt to shield him from anxiety and fear. These parents sincerely feel that they are rendering a service to the child — that he should be allowed to live his remaining time as free from worry and concern as possible. They are certain that by assuming their prediagnosis behavior they are reaffirming to the child that he will be all right, and they are firm in the conviction that they can preserve the child in an anxiety-free state as long as they maintain this behavior. It has been found, however, that the parents' denial of the existence of anxiety in the child arises primarily from the enormity of the parents' own anxiety. They are so involved with the death taboo and their own fears and grief that they are blinded to those of the child.

The child does perceive the disguised and altered emotional climate; his parents' attitude of intense concern is not concealed from him. The child possesses a remarkable awareness of the gravity of the situation. He knows that his condition is deteriorating — he has less energy, less appetite, and less enthusiasm. Vernick and Karon contend that it is ludicrous even to entertain the thought that the child might not know that he is seriously ill [41]. Solnit states that even when the parents make a deliberate attempt to shield a child from the truth, "children invariably sense what is happening to them" [40]. Waechter found that children express this knowledge through an increase in generalized anxiety [45].

A child in this situation is in a precarious position. He knows that he cannot speak with his parents concerning his fears and anxieties. Their evasiveness only tends to heighten his insecurity. In his unhappiness he may turn to his nurse for understanding and support. The nurse is thus in a crucial position. Because of his or her closeness to the child, the nurse has two options: to afford the child with a fatal illness an opportunity for emotional release, or to reinforce the death taboo by refusal to acknowledge the existence of the child's awareness of his impending death.

The purpose of this chapter is to lend support to the nurse's first option. Nurses must recognize their responsibility to the fatally ill child. They must become aware of the psychological needs of fatally ill children and provide a means of communication through which an emotional release may be obtained. It would be relatively easy to find a substantial excuse to follow a route of avoidance. Should nurses avail themselves of the opportunity for escape, however, the results for the child would be disastrous. As stated by Gullo [15],

It is only by facing the psychological as well as the physical suffering of such a person that the nurse can hope to give the type of help required by the terminally ill.... This "complete terminal care" may pose a burden to the nurse's time and psyche, but this is also her challenge as a professional committed to the highest standards of nursing.

The specific role of the nurse in the care of the fatally ill child is only now undergoing examination, and there is a noticeable lack of information about it in the literature. Quint stresses the need for personalized nursing care designed to meet the psychosocial needs of any patient, child or adult [35]. She suggests that this requires a provision for continuity of care, the opportunity for the patient to participate actively in his care, and the promotion of confidence and

trust in the nurse. Quint admits, however, that attention
to the psychological needs of the patient is an area that is
usually neglected [36]. She states that in large part this is
due to the reluctance of the nurse to communicate with
the fatally ill patient. Without communication it is difficult
to discern the patient's individual psychological needs.
Verwoerdt [42, 43] suggests that communication with a
fatally ill patient be directed toward three levels of understanding: (1) the meaning of the illness and its symptoms
to the patient, (2) the patient's awareness of and psychological reactions to the illness, and (3) the difficulties, fears,
and anxieties the patient experiences as a result of his
awareness and psychological reactions.

As stated, the reluctance of the nurse to communicate
with the dying child usually is based on her own inhibitions
concerning death. Also, many a nurse's fear of communication has focused on the question: "To tell or not to tell?"
As suggested, this question is irrelevant — the child knows.
The nurse must acknowledge the child's awareness. There
is one qualifying point, however. Specifically *what* the child
knows is dependent upon his age, stage of development, and
level of concept formation. His fears and anxieties are con-
tingent upon these factors. Therefore in order to determine
the particular psychological needs of a fatally ill child the
nurse must first understand the child's concept of death at
different stages.

The Child's Concept of Death

We shall consider the concepts of death in both healthy
children and ill children.

Healthy Children
One of the first definitive studies concerning the concept
of death in healthy children was that conducted by Nagy
[30]. Nagy divides the child's concept formation into three
stages. The first stage encompasses birth through the age
of five years. During this period the child does not acknowledge death as an irreversible state and continues to attribute
lifelike characteristics to dead persons. Two variations of
this thought are possible: (1) the child views death as a
departure, a going away, or a sleep and thus totally denies
the finality of death; or (2) the child recognizes physical
death but cannot distinguish it from life and considers it
temporary. The second stage of concept formation includes
children from age five to age nine. In this period the child
personifies death. Death may be envisioned as the dead
person himself or as a separate person (i.e., ghost, skeleton,
or bogeyman). Dying is thought of as a punishment for
wrongdoing, and the child associates it with evil, darkness,
and nighttime. In this second stage the child demonstrates
an increasing sense of reality, as he does acknowledge the
existence of death. But because this acknowledgment is so
upsetting, the child displaces the thought onto a person
other than himself; thus, death becomes personified. The
third stage of concept formation begins after the age of nine.
It is at this point that the child begins to envision death as
biologically based and as an inevitable occurrence. Nagy
concludes by stating that concealment of death from any
fatally ill child is not possible and should not be attempted.

Kastenbaum agrees in most part with Nagy's conceptual
framework. He describes the sequence of thought the child
follows in developing the concept "I will die" [18].

1. I am an individual with a life of my own, a personal existence.
2. I belong to a class of beings one of whose attributes is mortality.
3. Using the intellectual process of logical deduction, I must arrive at the conclusion that my personal death is a certainty.
4. There are many possible causes of my death, and these causes might operate in many different combinations; although I might evade or escape one particular cause, I cannot evade all causes.
5. My death will occur in the future. By future I mean a time-to-live that has not yet elapsed.
6. But I do not know when in the future my death will occur. The event is certain; the timing is uncertain.
7. Death is a final event. My life ceases. This means that I will never again experience, think, or act, at least as a human being on this earth.
8. Accordingly, death is the ultimate separation of myself from the world.

Kastenbaum asserts that the rapidity with which a child formulates these concepts varies among individual children but that predictions can be made, based on Nagy's framework, as to the expected level of comprehension.

Adler reported on Anthony's study with children aged three to nine [1]. Anthony found that no child under age eight had more than a very limited concept of death usually referring to some extraneous aspect of it (e.g., a coffin). Anthony also found two types of death anxiety in children: *chronic* death anxiety — a vague, indescribable fear in children up to five years of age — and *critical* death anxiety — a specific, describable fear in older children due to the realization of their own mortality.

Gartley and Bernasconi reported on a study of sixty Roman Catholic children [11]. (The variable of a constant religion may introduce a bias and thus place the results in question if applied to a larger population.) In the children aged five years and five months to six years and four months they found some giving of lifelike characteristics to the dead, unstructured and flexible concepts, death viewed as a remote idea and not perceived as something that could happen to them, death conceptualized in concrete terms (e.g., a coffin), and the absence of a death fear. Children aged six years and six months to seven years and five months were found to believe that heaven is a place from which there is no return, heaven is a restrictive place in which God replaces the parents in dictating rules, and that death is remote and in the distant future. Children aged seven years and five months to eight years and four months were found to believe in heaven and hell and to realize that death could be an immediate possibility for them. Children aged eight years and five months to nine years and eight months began to make a distinction between body and soul. They realized that death could be sudden and painful. Children aged nine years and six months and older were found to be much more reticent in speaking about death but in general followed Nagy's description of the third conceptual stage.

McIntire et al. investigated the concept of death in children aged five to eighteen [26] and found that in their minds death was most often associated with violence. In the age range of thirteen to sixteen, 60 percent of those interviewed felt there would be a spiritual continuation after death, 20 percent thought the dead would retain powers of cognition, and 20 percent visualized death as final.

In another study, Kastenbaum [19] found that the teen-ager viewed death as associated with old age and disease. The teenager felt that since much time would transpire before he became "old," he needn't be concerned about death in the present. Thus such thoughts were quickly dismissed.

Several additional studies were found to support the original ideas of Nagy concerning the concept of death in the healthy child [2, 6, 7, 16, 22, 27, 32, 44, 46]. All divide the child's concept formation into three general stages of approximately the same age and agree with the following summary: zero to five years – denial of death as personal reality; six to nine years – acceptance of death as personal reality, but vague ideas concerning the process of dying and the meaning of death; ten years and older – acceptance of personal death, more abstract, adult-like conceptualization of dying and death.

Ill Children
The concept of death in ill and dying children has been examined by various researchers. Richmond and Waisman [39] found that children with cancer rarely express overt concern about death. The children they talked to seemed to have an attitude of passivity and resignation which tended to increase with the progression of the disease. "Even among the adolescents, who intellectually may know much about cancer, the question concerning diagnosis and possibility of death usually was not raised as it often is by the adult patient. Our suspicion is that this does not reflect an unawareness but rather represents an attempt at repres-sion psychologically of the anxiety concerning death" [39].

Lourie feels that the "resignation" described by Richmond and Waisman is actually a cachexia and not a true representation of the child's attitudes toward death [24]. Vernick and Karon also disagree with the idea of passive resignation. They state that "every child who is lying in bed gravely ill is worrying about dying and is eager to have someone help him talk about it" [41, p. 395]. They stress that it is essential for the adult caregivers to structure an environment in which the child feels free to communicate.

Natterson and Knudson reported on a study of thirty-three fatally ill children [31]. They obtained the following results: age zero to five years – fear of separation predominates; age five to ten years – fear of procedures (e.g., mutilation) predominates; age ten years and older – fear of death predominates and is "urgent, pervasive, and persistent" [31]. Common behavioral manifestations included anxiety, depression, and withdrawal.

Morrissey studied fifty children with leukemia to determine the presence of a death anxiety [28]. He found that the anxiety was present mostly when the child was older. It was handled in one of three ways: (1) younger children expressed anxiety symbolically and physiologically, (2) older boys tended to act out, and (3) older girls tended to become depressed.

Waechter studied sixty-four fatally ill children between the ages of six and ten [45]. She found that even though the child was not directly told of his prognosis, he exhibited considerable preoccupation with death in fantasy. The child demonstrated feelings of loneliness and isolation, loss of control, and an inability to structure his psychological or physical environment. Waechter also found that although the child did possess a death anxiety, it was not overtly expressed. She proposes that the questions and concerns be dealt with as honestly and openly as possible. "Understanding acceptance of the child's fears and conveyance of permission to discuss any aspect of his illness may decrease these feelings of isolation, alienation and the sense that his illness is too terrible to discuss" [45, p. 18].

Easson, in a recent publication on the dying child, examines the child's understanding of death at various age levels [8]. At four years the child responds to changes in his body. Also, pain and fear may become conditioned responses to the approach of a white-coated person. At four to five years the child responds to the significance of his diagnosis. Although this comprehension varies with intellect, by this age most children know what "cancer," "leukemia," "tumor," and so forth represent. At five to seven years, Easson states the child responds to the significance of the prognosis. The child is able to conceptualize "time" and "future" and thus may become very anxious as he realizes the full significance of his prognosis. At six to seven years the child responds to the change in his role and social relationships. That is, as the child progresses through the stages of dying, he begins to acknowledge the changing status of his relationships with his parents, siblings, peers, hospital personnel, and others. Easson states that even at this relatively early age the child learns not to talk about his death, as it upsets those around him. Consequently he becomes isolated.

Psychological Needs of the Fatally Ill Child

It is evident from the preceding literature that the fatally ill child may have a great variety of psychological needs. In general these needs may be divided into three major areas: (1) overall emotional needs (needs which are common to all children, regardless of health status), (2) needs arising from the child's reaction to his illness and hospitalization, and (3) needs arising from his concept of death.

Overall Emotional Needs
According to Raths [38] needs common to all children include:

the need for love and affection
the need for achievement
the need for belonging
the need for self-respect
the need to be free from deep feelings of guilt
the need to be free from deep feelings of fear
the need for economic security
the need for understanding of self

It is readily apparent that each of these needs assumes increased significance in relation to the fatally ill child. Because of his altered routine and decreased contact with significant others, the fatally ill child is much less likely to be successful in achieving a level of positive equilibrium in satisfying these needs. It is thus essential that the nurse not lose sight of the fact that this particular fatally ill patient is a child, first and always. As such, he requires assistance with even the most common of needs.

Needs Arising from the Child's Reaction
to Illness and Hospitalization
As discussed, the child may harbor feelings of guilt and
blame for "bad behavior" or similar wrongdoing. He may
view his illness as a consequence of an inappropriate action.
Hospitalization may symbolize punishment. There is a loss
of constant contact with the parents and with siblings,
peers, pets, and favorite objects. The child requires considerable psychological help. His needs include support,
love, attention, understanding, approval, security, friend-
ship, compassion, acknowledgment, empathy, behavioral
limits, self-control, and discipline.

Needs Arising from the Child's Concept of Death
It has been found that a fatally ill child does have some
conceptualization of death. Furthermore he usually does
have a death anxiety. The specific definition of this death
anxiety varies with several factors: the child's age, maturity,
level of cognitive processes, diagnosis, prognosis, level of
awareness, relationship with parents, relationship with hospital personnel, religious affiliation, and association with
other dying children, and with the amount of self-expression
encouraged in the child. The presence of this death anxiety
can yield many psychological reactions, such as frustrations,
fears, anxieties, isolation, passivity, regression, and withdrawal. It has been shown, however, that the child is left
to his own devices to cope with this situation. The parents
and staff are too entangled in the death taboo to communicate with the child. Lowenberg discusses how this isolated
coping may yield either adaptive behavior (working through

problems) or maladaptive behavior (denying or avoiding problems) and feels that most frequently the result will be maladaptation [25]. Behavior indicative of this includes hostility, avoidance, inappropriate affect, psychosomatic symptoms, isolation, self-punitive feelings, and fantasizing.

In reviewing the many psychological needs of the fatally ill child it becomes apparent that there is one main need that encompasses and subsumes the remaining needs: that is, the need for a means of communication through which an emotional release may be achieved. The child has an overabundance of emotions aroused by his illness, hospitalization, and impending death. He may suffer psychologically from the severance of the communication lines with the parents and the staff. The child is in a precarious isolated position on an island, so overwhelmed and overcome by the turn of events in his life that he is in danger of sinking. Each of the many psychological needs brings with it a variety of emotions. When there is such a multitude of needs, the child may be totally surrounded by his thoughts, fears, and anxieties. High levels of anxiety may prohibit the child from any semblance of normal functioning. He may become immobilized and incapacitated.

The child must be enabled to understand, reduce to a manageable size, and overcome his fears and anxieties. Frequently the child turns to the nurse for this assistance and she must be ready to acknowledge this often silent request for help. She must be perceptive of his psychological needs. She must make an in-depth examination of her own role in relation to the death taboo. The nurse must overcome her reluctance to acknowledge the child's status overtly and must dissipate the hesitation she experiences when communicating with the child. Evasiveness, false cheerfulness, and superficiality must be replaced by openness, honesty, responsiveness, and acceptance of the child.

It is the responsibility of the nurse to take up this challenge. It is she who must provide the child with a convenient and acceptable outlet for emotional release. This outlet must afford the child an opportunity for self-expression, direct or indirect. It must be a means through which the child can express all his emotions positive and negative. It must provide a feeling of safety and security, so that the child need not fear adult reprisal for the revelation of forceful, negativistic feelings. Once expressed, these feelings must be dealt with in a manner that is beneficial to the child. Trust, faith, relief, security, and happiness are to be promoted.

Is there such a method, device, tool, or outlet available to the nurse? Fortunately, yes. Play, especially therapeutic play, meets the stated requirements.

Play
Why is it that play may be used as an opportunity for communication and emotional release? There are two main reasons. First, play is what communication authorities refer to as a *universal*. It is a mode of communication that cuts across many barriers. It is a common bond — it has similar traits and characteristics in most childhood orientations. It is not impeded by a lack of language skills. It does not require extensive training nor large investments of time or money. It is understandable to a wide variety of persons

of different ages. In sum, play knows no cultural, ethnic, racial, religious, financial, or other such boundaries.

Second, play is the natural means of communication for the child. Caplan and Caplan state that play is "all-pervasive, extraordinary, and supremely serious" [5]. It is the child's way of life. It provides a chance for the child to experience some control and mastery over his environment, in which he is usually the dependent one. Play is an intensely personal and voluntary activity. The child can determine which parts of the outside world he will tackle, comprehend, and assimilate and which parts he will temporarily reject and ignore. Play offers the child a free choice of action. Therefore he can make mistakes without fearing verbal or physical reprisals. Play provides an "inside world" where reality and fantasy are equally admissible. Play affords the child an opportunity to integrate social processes. It is the practice session for identifying, comprehending, and coping with feelings in the reality situation. Play is dynamic, free, vitalizing, and essential to the life of the child.

Play Therapy
Various psychologists and psychiatrists have realized the value of incorporating play into their work with troubled children. Melanie Klein and Anna Freud were among the first to theorize the benefits to be gained from establishing play as an integral component of child psychoanalysis [10]. Anna Freud points out that it is unreasonable to expect a child to assume a recumbent position and verbally communicate the nature of his problem as an adult might. The child does not have the cognitive powers necessary to

formulate a clear identification of the problem. The child
does not have the language skills necessary to verbalize the
problem. Also, the child is not capable of free association
(a major tool in psychoanalysis). While speech is the mode
of communication in the adult, play is the mode of communication in the child. Play is a much more natural means for
the child to use to communicate to the sensitive adult. Klein
states that just as she would examine the adult's spoken
word for meaning, she would search for meaning in the
child's actions. Both Klein and Freud conclude that the
child expresses his inner thoughts and emotions in his play.

Axline describes the process of unstructured, nondirective play therapy [3], which is based on this assumption
that play is the child's natural medium for self-expression.
This type of play therapy extends an opportunity to the
child to "play out" his feelings of fright, anger, hostility,
isolation, resentment, aggression, confusion, and so forth.
Nondirective play therapy is also based on the assumption
that "the individual has within himself, not only the ability
to solve his own problems satisfactorily, but also a growth
impulse that makes mature behavior more satisfying than
immature behavior" [3, p. 15]. Thus, this type of play
therapy extends to the child the opportunity to "experience
growth under the most favorable conditions" and to gain
increasing insight, self-control, and mastery [3, pp. 73–74].

During a play therapy session, a child is taken to a playroom equipped with various kinds of toys. The child is
free to pursue any object of interest and to play with it in
the manner he desires. The more uninhibited the child is
in action or verbal expression, the more data the therapist

can collect on which to extrapolate meaning. The freedom
with which the child experiences this opportunity for play
(and thus for learning and for growth) is directly attributable
to the atmosphere and environment created by the therapist
in the playroom. If the child senses that the therapist is
permissive, encouraging, and accepting, the child will be
increasingly prompted to allow his true desires and feelings
to dictate his actions and words. If the child senses that
the therapist is rigid, directive, or punitive, the child's inner
feelings will be carefully guarded and submerged. Axline
suggests that there are eight basic principles which a therapist should utilize in attempting to create an appropriate
play therapy environment [3, pp. 73–74]:

1. The therapist must develop a warm, friendly relationship with
   the child, in which good rapport is established as soon as possible.
2. The therapist accepts the child exactly as he is.
3. The therapist establishes a feeling of permissiveness in the relationship so that the child is free to express his feelings completely.
4. The therapist is alert to recognize the feelings the child is expressing and reflects those feelings back to him in such a manner that
   he gains insight into his behavior.
5. The therapist maintains a deep respect for the child's ability to
   solve his own problems if given an opportunity to do so. The responsibility to make choices and to institute change is the child's.
6. The therapist does not attempt to direct the child's actions or
   conversation in any manner. The child leads the way; the therapist
   follows.
7. The therapist does not attempt to hurry the therapy. It is a
   gradual process and is recognized as such by the therapist.
8. The therapist establishes only those limitations that are necessary
   to anchor the therapy to the world of reality and to make the
   child aware of his responsibility in the relationship.

Once the benefits to be gained by play therapy were well demonstrated and substantiated, the technique was examined by various researchers to determine if a similar method might be devised within the realm of nursing care. Although it was found that play therapy requires the supervision of a psychologist, psychiatrist, or psychiatric nurse clinician, it was also found that with the introduction of several basic revisions the technique was adaptable as a tool for the professional nurse. The revised technique — therapeutic play — retains as its primary goal the provision to the child of an opportunity for self-expression through the medium of play.

Therapeutic Play
Therapeutic play is based upon the unstructured, nondirective form of play therapy, with modifications to allow the nurse to function as the therapist. As in play therapy the focus is on assisting the child to help himself by providing a comfortable mode of communication. The nurse, although nondirective, does not assume a passive role. She must be an active listener who consistently offers acceptance and permissiveness. She is empathetic, sensitive, interested, and alert. She must respect the child and treat him honestly and fairly. She must be familiar with growth and development, the child's personal history, and his familial resources. The nurse stresses kindness, understanding, patience, and steadiness. She maintains a liking for the child and exhibits faith and confidence in the child's ability to handle his problems.

It is important for the nurse to establish a feeling of

acceptance of the child in the therapeutic play session. The child should be encouraged to relax and be himself. An atmosphere of freedom and permissiveness is highly desirable. The child should become accustomed to assuming an independent, self-directed role. Only those limitations that are necessary for safety and realistic boundaries are to be established.

As in play therapy the child is offered a variety of toys during a therapeutic play session. Depending upon the available facilities, he may be taken to a special playroom or toys may be taken to his bedside. Juenker [17] suggests that dramatic play props such as dolls, hand puppets, and family-life figures are useful for creative, imaginative, and expressive play. Aggressive toys like drums, cymbals, and squirt guns are conducive to the expression of hostility and anger. Regressive toys like a nursing bottle and a baby blanket are frequently used for expression of "babyish" feelings. Toys that provide free creative expression (crayons and construction paper, finger paints and paper) may be offered. Constructive toys also may be included, such as building blocks and modeling clay. Age-appropriate toys are important. A preschool-aged child may especially enjoy dress-up clothes, whereas a school-aged child may enjoy a game of scribbage. A child who has intense feelings about his illness, hospitalization, or impending death may eagerly seize an opportunity for play with doctor, nurse, and patient figures. Clean syringes are favorites, and a stethoscope, tongue blade, cotton swab, thermometer, miniature bed, oxygen mask, intravenous equipment, and so forth, are very conducive for play.

After providing the child with a variety of toys the nurse acts in a nondirective manner. She does not suggest which toys to use nor which activities to pursue; the selection is the child's prerogative. It is also up to the child to set the pace of the therapeutic play session. It may be a gradual process; the nurse should make no attempt to rush the child.

The reflective technique is an important component of the therapeutic play session. For example, one nine-year-old fatally ill child drew a picture of a little girl with a big frown on her face and stated, "The little girl is sad. She is going away and misses her mommy." The nurse responded, "Oh, I see. The little girl is very sad because she is going away and she misses her mommy." This reflection assured the child that the nurse was listening and that she was interested. It also encouraged the child to continue playing. Petrillo and Sanger caution, however, that the nurse should reflect only the verbal expressions of the child in a therapeutic play session [33]. To go beyond the reflection of verbal expressions is to enter the domain of play therapy.

Thus it can be seen that there are various similarities between play therapy and therapeutic play. Both techniques propose to achieve an emotional release for the child by providing him with the opportunity for self-expression. One of the major differences between the two techniques, however, is the handling of the child's feelings and expressions. In play therapy the therapist reflects the child's feelings *and* expressions. The therapist interprets and explains these to the child. In therapeutic play the nurse reflects *only* the child's expressions and carefully determines if and when it is appropriate to go beyond these to the underlying feelings. She does *not* interpret or explain either the expressions or the possible feelings behind them. To do so would be inappropriate, considering the nurse's limited preparation in psychiatry. The accompanying chart outlines a comparison of various other differences between play therapy and therapeutic play.

Comparison of Play Therapy and Therapeutic Play

Play Therapy	Therapeutic Play
Primary goal To provide an opportunity to the child for self-expression	*Primary goal* To provide an opportunity to the child for self-expression
Secondary goal To assist the *child* to gain insight into his behaviors, expressions, and feelings	*Secondary goal* To assist the *nurse* to gain insight into the child's behaviors, expressions, and feelings
Therapist Psychiatrist, psychologist, or psychiatric nurse clinician	*Therapist* Professional nurse
Client Emotionally disturbed, neurotic, or psychotic child	*Client* Any hospitalized child
Environment Specially prepared playroom	*Environment* Hospital playroom, bedside, or any convenient area
Length Usually one hour	*Length* Usually fifteen to forty-five minutes
Duration Usually several months	*Duration* Varies from one time only to daily during hospitalization
Reflective technique Reflection of verbal expressions and nonverbal feelings	*Reflective technique* Reflections of verbal expressions only
Interpretation Significant behaviors, expressions, and/or feelings interpreted to the child to promote insight	*Interpretation* *No* interpretations made to child
Main proponents Axline [3], Moustakas [29]	*Main proponents* Petrillo and Sanger [33], Plank [34]

Within the realm of nursing therapeutic play can do much toward enhancing communication with the fatally ill child. As the child becomes more familiar with the process of therapeutic play, feelings of safety and security in the play environment are strengthened and trust in the nurse is fostered. The child relaxes and becomes more comfortable with the use of the toys. He begins increasingly to take advantage of the opportunity for communication.

The alert nurse may elicit clues from the play as to the child's thoughts or concerns.

Child A, age nine, with leukemia, was playing with a group of family puppets. The child enacted a story about a little boy who "got sick and had to go to the hospital to get some blood."

The nurse may also be able to discern areas of misinformation or confusion which would benefit from intervention.

Child B, age four and a half, with leukemia (in reverse isolation), drew a picture of a little boy who had "bad, bad blood so they put him in a room and shut the door — SLAM! — and no one wanted to see him."

Areas of deep concern or fear (i.e., death) may be revealed in a therapeutic play session.

Child C, age eight, with renal failure, drew a picture of an airplane superimposed over a building. He told the story that "there were people on the plane going on a vacation — the plane crashed into the building — all the people died."

Repetition of a theme in therapeutic play may be indicative of an especially persistent or deep-rooted concern.

In another session Child C drew a picture of a boat with fish swimming above it. He told the story that "the boat was going on a weekend fishing trip — the boat crashed into a rock and got a hole and sank — all the people died."

Separation anxieties are frequently expressed.

Child D, age five, with medulloblastoma, drew in the lefthand corner of the page a picture of a large building with a small frowning person inside. Off to the right was a very small house. The child stated, "The boy in the hospital is sad — he is far away from his house."

Feelings of repression, confinement, and punishment may be elicited.

Child E, age seven, with renal failure, drew a picture of a little girl strapped flat by thick ropes which were attached to a large machine. The child stated, "Two times a week the girl is tied to the machine for a long time."

A child's preoccupation with his illness may be revealed to the nurse.

Child F, age thirteen, with osteogenic sarcoma, drew a picture of a girl with a left leg enlarged in the same location as her own tumor.

The influence of the environment on the integrity of the child may be demonstrated.

Child G, age twelve, with systemic lupus erythematosus, drew a picture of a child lying in bed. The child was surrounded by a heart monitor, IVs, oxygen tank, and other equipment. The child was very small in relation to the large and abundant pieces of equipment.

Fears of loss of self-identity often are revealed.

Child H, age four, a girl with cystic fibrosis, drew a picture of a child sitting in a bed with a mist-tent-like device over the bed. The child stated, "She will get all wet in there and will look like a boy."

The desires and wishes of the child are not infrequently found.

Child I, age ten, with leukemia, drew a picture of a boy at a baseball game. He muttered under his breath, "I wish I was there."

As these examples demonstrate, a wide variety of thoughts, feelings, concerns, and anxieties may be elicited from the child during a therapeutic play session. It is the responsibility of the nurse to utilize these expressions of self (verbal or nonverbal) effectively. Communication with the fatally ill child is complete only when three requirements are met: (1) provision of opportunity for communication through therapeutic play, (2) elicitation of clues from the play behavior as to the child's thoughts, anxieties, and needs, and (3) utilization of these clues to meet the needs of the child.

The following seven-step process* is suggested as a method by which the professional nurse may utilize clues from the

*Reprinted with permission from the October 1974 issue of *Nursing '74*, copyright 1974 by Intermed Communications, Inc., Jenkintown, Pa.

child in planning pertinent nursing care to meet the child's individual needs [14].

Observe   Observe the child's play. (Is he happy or angry? Is he extroverted and free, or is he introverted and precise? Is he concentrating heavily or does his attention wander?)

Examine   Examine the play behavior for its overt content. (Who does the child talk about? What is the environment? What objects of importance are included?)

Analyze   Analyze the play behavior for its covert meaning. (What does the child mean? What inner feelings might he be expressing? What is currently happening to the child that might correlate with or help explain the child's comments and behaviors?)

Validate   Validate your conclusion about the meaning of the child's comments and play behavior with another nurse. (For example, "Mark drew a picture of an airplane during his play. He said that the plane crashed and all the passengers died. Currently, Mark is undergoing renal dialysis. I think his picture means that he is afraid he is going to die. What do you think?")

Determine   Determine if outside professional assistance is needed to understand the child's comments and behavior. (Did the second nurse validate your conclusions? If not, do you need assistance from the house psychologist or psychiatrist? Can the psychiatric nurse clinician provide insight?)

Plan   Plan pertinent nursing intervention to meet the need expressed by the child. (For example, Jody drew a picture of a jail-like crib indicating that she felt that she was being punished — "put in jail." Appropriate intervention would be to talk with the child about the reasons for hospitalization, feelings that the child might be experiencing, the role of the nurse in helping the child, and so on.)

Evaluate   Evaluate the effectiveness of the therapeutic play process. (Effectiveness will depend on how well you have identified and responded to the child's concerns.)

Not effective — If a need has been incorrectly identified, and thus the nursing activities have not been pertinent, the nurse may expect to see a continuation or increase in the clue-giving behavior in subsequent therapeutic play sessions. A careful re-assessment of the clues should be made to identify the need accurately.

Partially effective — If a need has been correctly identified, but the nursing activities have not been helpful to the child in meeting the need, the nurse may expect to see a continuation of the clue-giving behavior in subsequent therapeutic play sessions. Planning of alternative nursing actions should be initiated.

Effective — If a need has been correctly identified and the nursing activities have been appropriate in fulfilling the need, the nurse may expect to see a decrease or cessation of the clue-giving behavior in subsequent therapeutic play sessions. Intervention should be continued until the nurse feels the need no longer exists.

Used in this manner, the therapeutic play process becomes an invaluable tool as a means of communication and emotional release for the fatally ill child. In addition, it is of great assistance in providing insight into the complex and isolated world of the fatally ill child.

Summary and Conclusion
A review of the status of the dying child has been conducted from a nursing perspective. It has been found that the child

has many psychological needs arising from his illness, hospitalization, and impending death. It also has been found that the child desires meaningful communication with his parents and the staff concerning these needs but usually is denied this communication because of the involvement of the parents and the staff with the death taboo. Consequently the child is left to his own devices to cope with the situation. If the child is overwhelmed by his feelings, anxieties, and fears, maladaptive behavioral changes may be precipitated. The fatally ill child experiences a pervasive, omnipresent, crucial need for communication through which an emotional release may be obtained. The professional nurse is in a particularly suitable position to help the child by providing a safe, acceptable outlet for the release of emotions. Therapeutic play may be used (1) to provide a comfortable means of communication by which the child may obtain an emotional release, (2) to provide insight into the child's thoughts, feelings, and behavior, and (3) to plan pertinent nursing care to meet the individual needs of the fatally ill child.

The nursing profession must be aware of the consequences that result from the perpetuation of the death taboo. Vigorous steps must be undertaken and continued to demonstrate its inherent fallacies and to prevent its propagation. Within the acute care facilities, workshops, and in-service educational programs should be provided for the nurses to disengage their concepts of terminal care from the last remaining grasp of the mid-Victorian period. Within the educational facilities, innovative and creative nurse-teachers must continually construct and improve the curriculum to provide a sound, comprehensive, and operational conceptual framework of the dying child. Responsive and sensitive professional nurses must be educated to utilize this conceptual framework in planning care for the dying child. Full responsibility must be assumed for the entire care of the child, both physical and psychological. Then, and only then, can we be assured that the dying child's total needs will be met.

References

1. Adler, C. S. The meaning of death to children. *Ariz. Med.* 3:266, 1969.
2. Alexander, I., and Adlerstein, A. Affective responses to the concept of death in a population of children and early adolescents. *J. Genet. Psychol.* 93:167, 1958.
3. Axline, V. *Play Therapy.* New York: Ballantine, 1969.
4. Bowlby, J. Grief and mourning in infancy and early childhood. *Psychoanal. Study Child* 15:9, 1960.
5. Caplan, F., and Caplan, T. *The Power of Play.* New York: Doubleday, 1973.
6. Caprio, F. S. A study of some psychological reactions during pre-pubescence to the idea of death. *Psychiatr. Q.* 24:495, 1950.
7. Childers, P., and Wimmer, M. Concept of death in early childhood. *Child Dev.* 42:1299, 1971.
8. Easson, W. M. *The Dying Child — The Management of the Child or Adolescent Who is Dying.* Springfield, Ill.: Thomas, 1970.
9. Feifel, H., and Farberow, N. (Eds.) *Taboo Topics.* New York: Atherton, 1963.
10. Freud, A. *The Psycho-Analytic Treatment of the Child.* New York: Schocken, 1964.
11. Gartley, W., and Bernasconi, M. The concept of death in children. *J. Genet. Psychol.* 110:71, 1967.

12. Geis, D. P. Mothers' perceptions of care given their dying children. *Am. J. Nurs.* 65:105, 1965.
13. Gorer, G. The Pornography of Death. In Stein, M., and Vidich, A. (Eds.), *Identity and Anxiety.* New York: Free Press of Glencoe, 1960.
14. Green, C. S. Understanding children's needs through therapeutic play. *Nursing '74* 4(10):30, 1974.
15. Gullo, S. V. Thanatology: The study of death and the care of the dying. *Bedside Nurse* 5:11, 1972.
16. Howarth, R. The psychiatry of terminal illness. *Proc. R. Soc. Med.* 65:1039, 1972.
17. Juenker, D. Play as a Tool of the Nurse. In Steele, S. (Ed.), *Nursing Care of the Child with Long-Term Illness.* New York: Appleton-Century-Crofts, 1971.
18. Kastenbaum, R. The Child's Understanding of Death. In E. A. Grollman (Ed.), *Explaining Death to Children.* Boston: Beacon, 1967, p. 93.
19. Kastenbaum, R. Time and Death in Adolescence. In Feifel, H. (Ed.), *The Meaning of Death.* New York: McGraw-Hill, 1959.
20. Kneisl, C. R. Thoughtful care for the dying. *Am. J. Nurs.* 68:550, 1968.
21. Kübler-Ross, E. *On Death and Dying.* New York: Macmillan, 1969.
22. Lascari, A. D. The family and the dying child. *Med. Times* 97:207, 1969.
23. Lindemann, E. Symptomatology and management of acute grief. *Am. J. Psychiatry* 101:141, 1944.
24. Lourie, R. S. The pediatrician and the handling of terminal illness. *Pediatrics* 32:477, 1963.
25. Lowenberg, J. S. The coping behaviors of fatally-ill adolescents and their parents. *Nurs. Forum* 9:269, 1970.
26. McIntire, M., Angle, C. R., and Struempler, L. T. The concept of death in Midwestern children and youth. *Am. J. Dis. Child.* 123:527, 1972.
27. Miya, T. M. The child's perception of death. *Nurs. Forum* 11:214, 1972.

28. Morrissey, J. R. Death Anxiety in Children with Fatal Illness. In Parad, H. J. (Ed.), *Crisis Intervention: Selected Readings.* New York: Family Service Association, 1965.

29. Moustakas, C. E. *Psychotherapy with Children — The Living Relationship.* New York: Ballantine, 1970.

30. Nagy, M. The Child's View of Death. In Feifel, H. (Ed.), *The Meaning of Death.* New York: McGraw-Hill, 1959, pp. 79–98.

31. Natterson, J. M., and Knudson, A. G. Observations concerning fear of death in fatally-ill children and their mothers. *Psychol. Med.* 22:456, 1960, p. 460.

32. Pacyna, D. A. Response to a dying child. *Nurs. Clin. North Am.* 5:421, 1970.

33. Petrillo, M., and Sanger, S. *Emotional Care of Hospitalized Children.* Philadelphia: Lippincott, 1972.

34. Plank, E. N. *Working with Children in Hospitals.* Cleveland: Press of Case Western Reserve University, 1962.

35. Quint, J. C. Obstacles to helping the dying. *Am. J. Nurs.* 66:1568, 1966.

36. Quint, J. C. *The Nurse and the Dying Patient.* New York: Macmillan, 1967.

37. Quint, J. C., and Strauss, A. L. Nursing students, assignments, and dying patients. *Nurs. Outlook* 12:24, 1964.

38. Raths, L. E. *Meeting the Needs of Children: Creating Trust and Security.* Columbus, Ohio: Merrill, 1972, p. 25.

39. Richmond, J. B., and Waisman, H. A. Psychologic aspects of management of children with malignant diseases. *Am. J. Dis. Child.* 89:42, 1955, p. 43.

40. Solnit, A. J., and Provence, S. A. *Modern Perspectives in Child Development.* New York: International University Press, 1963, p. 222.

41. Vernick, J., and Karon, M. Who's afraid of death on a leukemia ward? *Am. J. Dis. Child.* 109:393, 1965.

42. Verwoerdt, A. *Communication with the Fatally-Ill.* Springfield, Ill.: Thomas, 1966.

43. Verwoerdt, A., and Wilson, R. Communication with fatally-ill patients — Tacit or explicit? *Am. J. Nurs.* 67:2307, 1967.

44. Von Hug-Hellmuth, H. The child's concept of death. *Psychoanal. Q.* 34:499, 1965.
45. Waechter, E. Death anxiety in children with fatal illness. Ph.D. diss., Stanford University, 1968.
46. Zeligs, R. Children's attitudes toward death. *Ment. Hygiene* 51:393, 1967.

Bibliography

Browning, M. H., and Lewis, E. P. (Eds.), *The Dying Patient: A Nursing Perspective.* New York: American Journal of Nursing, 1972.

Glaser, B. G., and Strauss, A. L. The social loss of dying patients. *Am. J. Nurs.* 64:119, 1964.

Hamovitch, M. B. *The Parent and the Fatally-Ill Child.* Los Angeles, Calif.: Delmar, 1964.

Jackson, N. A. A Child's Pre-occupation with Death. In *A.N.A. Clinical Sessions.* New York: Appleton-Century-Crofts, 1968, pp. 172–179.

Karon, M., and Vernick, J. An approach to the emotional support of fatally-ill children. *Clin. Pediatr.* 7:274, 1968.

Morse, J. The goal of life enhancement for a fatally-ill child. *Children* 17:63, 1970.

Noble, E. *Play and the Sick Child.* London: Faber, 1967.

Pratt, M. A. A Hospitalized Pre-school Child Copes With a Fatal Illness. In *A.N.A. Clinical Sessions.* New York: Appleton-Century-Crofts, 1968, pp. 190–198.

Schoenberg, B., Carr, A. C., Peretz, D., and Kutscher, A. H. (Eds.), *Psychosocial Aspects of Terminal Care.* New York: Columbia University Press, 1972.

Steele, S. Nursing Care of the Child with Terminal Illness. In Steele, S. (Ed.), *Nursing Care of the Child with Long-Term Illness.* New York: Appleton-Century-Crofts, 1971.

Winnicott, D. W. Playing: Its theoretical status in the clinical situation. *J. Psychoanal.* 49:591, 1968.

7. GROWING UP TO DYING: THE CHILD, THE PARENTS, AND THE NURSE

Claudine R. Gartner

Understanding the child's view of death and parents' reactions to the death of their child necessitates understanding the different stages of child development and how parents understand, relate to, and cope with the child at each particular developmental level. In this chapter we shall present the infant, child, and adolescent of various stages of development and discuss parents' reactions to the death of a child in the various age groups. The emphasis will be on the developmental tasks achieved by the young child and how the understanding of personality development will help the parents better to sustain and support him and themselves during the death and grieving process. Continued understanding of the older child and his developmental achievement will allow the parents to give him the base needed for the maturing process of growing up to dying.

"Growing up to dying" is what we are calling the developmental process the child must go through in order to die with dignity. The parents must understand the phases of development that the child is passing through to be able to assist him and to accept his death with dignity.

The nurse's understanding of the basic needs and developmental achievement of the child will provide a sound base for the supportive care of the child and his parents. Very simply, getting to know the child and his parents, gathering data, and objectively interpreting the data will help the nurse to give the care needed by each child and his parents at this particular time.

The Infant (Newborn to Four Months)
The act of dying is always a lonely act, but for the very young infant it is one of utter aloneness, since he cannot

gain psychological support and reassurance from caring people [4]. The developmental task that the infant is attempting to achieve is a sense of trust and security [5]. Trust can exist only in relation to someone or something. At this early age contact with a gentle, caring person who provides pleasant, satisfying experiences for the baby is necessary to lay the basis for trust. For the most part it is not difficult to develop a sense of trust in the young infant, since it hinges on feeding, fondling, fussing with, and favoring the infant. Most adult human beings respond to infants in such a way as to satisfy this basic need.

The newborn infant and the infant up to four months of age who are dying are overwhelmed by physical sensations. The pain, frustrations, tensions, and fears that they experience cause them to struggle valiantly against these sensations. The infant fights against death with all the strength that he possesses [4]. At this point, when the infant relates to people only through taste, touch, sound, and smell, the only comfort he can receive is through feeding, holding, cuddling, touching, and soothing sounds and voices. It is imperative that parents be allowed to hold their dying infant as much as possible and that the nurse assist them to provide whatever else can comfort the child. If the infant is able to retain food, this should be provided as often as feasible. The sucking process, the intake of food that satisfies hunger pangs, and the closeness of a person who gives warmth and bodily contact will give comfort to the infant. If the infant is being breastfed, this should be continued as long as possible. The mother may find it extremely painful and difficult emotionally to continue breastfeeding her

infant, since this closeness will only strengthen the emotional ties that will soon need to be severed. The nurse can
help the mother in performing this mothering task by stay-
ing with her to assist in the care of the infant should anything happen during the feeding period. She should stay
with the mother to provide the emotional support she
needs. The nurse can talk to the mother about the comfort
the baby derives from the nursing process and the mother's
warmth and closeness. This is an ideal time for the nurse
to help the mother express her feelings about her baby and
the impending death of the baby. She can help the mother
to identify which mothering tasks she is capable of performing for her child. If the infant is unable to take or retain
food, a pacifier should be used to satisfy the sucking need
as long as the sucking reflex is present.

Feeding is one tangible way to comfort the dying infant.
Other means of comfort are holding, rocking, and cuddling.
If the parents are hesitant about doing this, the nurse should
assure them that it is allowed. She should pick the infant
up and show parents how to hold the baby, then place it
in the mother's or father's arms, supporting them until they
do feel confident that they are holding the infant properly.
The nurse needs to explain the proper positioning of the
infant's head so he can breathe freely. If his head falls
forward, the airway may become obstructed. If the baby
is held up on the shoulder, care should be taken that nose
and mouth are free for breathing. If the parents are fearful of handling the baby because of equipment, instructions
should be given them. If the infant is getting intravenous
therapy, the parents should be shown how to handle the

baby and tubings. They should be shown the site of injection. The nurse should explain the importance of being careful not to dislodge the needle. She should assure the parents that they are competent to handle the baby without harming him. If the infant has a nasogastric tube or a gastrostomy tube, the reason for the tubings should be explained. Any special precautions regarding the equipment attached to the baby should be explained. The nurse should not leave the parents alone with their infant until she has established with certainty that they are confident and comfortable with the baby and any special attachments he might have.

Tactile stimulation is essential for proper growth and development of any child, and it should be continued for any dying infant. Touch puts the baby in contact with someone and provides comfort. Tactile stimulation can be accomplished while holding, rocking, cuddling, and feeding. It should also be a matter of concern when bathing the baby or when performing any other necessary treatments. Gentle actions in changing dressings or giving treatments will reduce anxiety in the infant. Rubbing the baby's body gently while bathing, rubbing with lotion after the bath, stroking the head or arm, letting the infant grasp and hold a finger are all ways of conveying tenderness, stimulation, and love. Care should be taken that overstimulation does not occur. The infant does need periods of undisturbed rest and relaxation. Bathing and tactile stimulation are other tasks that parents can perform for their infant. Again, the nurse must determine their readiness for these tasks. If the parents are eager and comfortable in holding their baby, they are usually ready to give other care. Other indications of readiness would be facial expressions of concern or eagerness when the nurse is bathing the baby, talking about how they bathed the baby at home and things they did during bath time, directly asking if they could bathe the baby, and demonstrating that they are fairly comfortable with feeding and with special equipment used in treating the infant. When any of these evidences of readiness are present, the nurse should assist the parents in the performance of this task for their infant. She should also make clear to them that bathing the baby every day is not necessary if it is disturbing or painful.

Auditory stimulation should be a matter of concern for the young infant as well as the older one. Harsh, loud, sudden crashing sounds should be kept at a minimum. The infant needs soft, soothing, reassuring voices and sounds to minimize his panic and fear. He needs one sound at a time to relate to. Many sounds or voices add to his confusion and frustration. Anyone who contacts the infant should be especially careful to use a soft, soothing voice and to talk to the infant as he is performing any care. The infant may become very apprehensive if things are done to him and no sound is connected with them. Auditory stimulation can be accomplished by singing softly, playing music boxes or radios, or using tapes of parents' voices singing or telling a story to their child. This approach may seem premature for the young infant, but the earlier purposeful auditory stimulation is begun, the more effective it is.

Visual stimulation should be begun as early as possible, to help the infant develop eye focus and to make him familiar with the world around him. Types of visual activities would be crib mobiles, different types and colors of toys, and faces of significant persons within range of the child's vision.

The main thing in the care of the dying young infant is to keep his development as normal as possible, thus keeping him as free as possible from frustration and panic. It is essential to the dying young infant that the caring tasks be performed for him with great tenderness and love. This usually can be accomplished best by parents who really know and love the child. The parents should be helped to perform these tasks with assurance and a certain amount of efficiency. I have worked with many parents who with minimal instruction were able to feed their infants by gavage feeding, change dressings, and administer treatments without any difficulty. The parents' greatest comfort when their infant is dying is to know that they have done all that they are capable of doing for him. The nurse must learn to assume the role of instructor, counselor, supporter, and reinforcer. She does not need to care for the infant, she needs to help the parents to do so.

The Older Infant (Four to Fifteen Months)
When the infant reaches the age of four to nine months, he is still attempting to achieve a sense of trust and security [5]. At this age he begins to respond to people and pleasant situations. He is especially adept at provoking favorable responses from his mother, and he shows fear and anxiety when people are different from his mother or the significant person in his life. He recognizes and feels pain and discom-

fort and demonstrates fear of treatments and unfamiliar procedures and surroundings.

At twelve to fifteen months of age the infant begins to develop a sense of autonomy [5]. He begins to perceive himself as a distinct individual and no longer fears that if mother goes away, he will cease to exist. He is beginning to want to be independent and yet needs guidance, external controls, and rewards. His personality has not yet advanced to the extent that he is able to exert inner control over his feelings, fears, and drives. He is still dependent on his parents to set limitations on his behavior, and he needs to know that when his anger or panic becomes uncontrollable and unbearable, they will soothe him and help him reorganize his defenses. He needs to know that the parents will be there to protect him against an unfamiliar and threatening world. The older infant needs the same care from his mother and father as the young infant does, but needs it even more desperately, as he is unable and unwilling to accept mothering care from anyone who has not previously been the focus of his life. He perceives his universe through the one who fulfills his needs.

The adverse effects on the infant of discontinuance of the parent-child relationship have been perceived in many cases in which parents have been too distraught or emotionally immobilized to visit or care for their children [7]. When learning that the child has a terminal illness, they leave him in the hospital and do not return until he is near death or dead. I have observed situations in which infants of six months and older were admitted to the hospital responding normally: smiling, looking around, cooing, eating, and enjoying any handling or fondling. Gradually these infants have become lethargic and quiet. Within several months they completely stop noting the environment, stop eating and sucking, stop cooing and smiling, and sob softly instead of crying. Generally they present withdrawn behavior, characteristic of the phase of despair of the separation anxiety process. Many parents and nurses are unaware of the fright and pain the young child experiences when he is abandoned by his parents. It is essential that nurses understand the child's reactions and try to interpret these to the parents. The nurse who assists parents in understanding their infant's needs and reactions will be helping them to achieve the first step in the process of growing up to accepting the death of their infant and helping their infant to die in comfort and security. The parents who understand how much their baby needs them will not stay away from him, although being with him may be painful for them.

The parents need to be helped to see how the infant takes on their feelings and reactions. The older infant needs all the specific care and stimulation that was indicated for the young infant, and this care should be provided with as much feeling of security and peaceful calm as possible. It is difficult to see how parents can be joyful when their infant is dying. However, if they can be emotionally supported when they are not with their infant, they may be able to assume this role when caring for him. The nurse should have a period with the parents before they are with the infant to let them express their concerns and grief in any way they wish. She can elicit responses by asking how they feel at this particular time, picking up cues and following through on them. She can tell them that if they feel like crying, they should cry; and if she feels like it, she should cry with them. She can tell the parents about the responses and reactions the infant has shown since their last visit. The nurse should try to find out the methods the parents have used to get a happy and favorable response from their infant and encourage them to continue this approach. If the parents frequently have a period of time with a supporting person, they will be able to mobilize their ego strength to continue being supportive to their child. With this kind of help they will not withdraw from the infant before he has died but will be able to comfort, care for, and convey their love to him.

Sudden Infant Death Syndrome

During the period from two weeks to one year of age (and occasionally up to the age of three years) there is the possibility of sudden infant death syndrome (SIDS) occurring. This is a distinct disease characterized by sudden, unexpected death during sleep. SIDS is the number one cause of death for infants up to one year of age. Approximately 10,000 babies die each year from this syndrome [1].

The typical picture of sudden infant death syndrome is that a normal, healthy, thriving baby is put to bed and found dead during the night or in the morning, usually in the same position as when put to bed. Seldom is there any evidence of a struggle. There is blood-tinged froth coming from the nose and mouth. The face or the back of the head are deep purple where blood has pooled. Urine and stool have been passed. Autopsy findings, which have been similar in most cases, include pulmonary congestion and edema, intrathoracic petechiae, and minor pharyngeal edema. The final event leading to the death is believed to be laryngospasm [1].

The suddenness of the child's death causes parental reactions that are not present in parents who know that their child is ill and is going to die. Parents of children who die from SIDS have no preparation and no time for anticipatory grief [2]. All the grieving process must be endured after the fact. After the initial shock is over, the main responses are guilt and self-blame. The parents blame themselves for not recognizing that the child was ill, for not checking the baby more frequently, for leaving a blanket in the crib, or for leaving the baby with a relative or babysitter. Besides coping with feelings of shock, loss, and blame, they have to go through the experience of getting a doctor or taking their baby to the emergency room to be pronounced dead. These parents need to be given much consideration and support from doctors and nurses. Rules, regulations, and paper procedures should be waived until parents are able to cope or until relatives arrive. There are few meaningful words of consolation at this time. Nonverbal empathy can be expressed by an arm around the shoulder, offering a glass of water, providing a comfortable, private place for the parents, letting them hold the baby if they wish to, allowing family members to stay with them, calling their minister if they desire, and any other small acts of human kindness that the nurse can think of.

The timing of a request for an autopsy is very important, as is an appropriate explanation of the need for it. Immediately after the death of the baby parents may not want to be concerned with consent for an autopsy. Some better time should be found to obtain their consent. Autopsies are necessary for continued research in the hope of finding the cause of this syndrome but are also important for the parents' peace of mind [2]. The findings on the autopsy will reassure them later that it was not their fault and there was nothing they could have done to prevent their child's death.

Parents who lose a child by SIDS need follow-up counseling. The nurse should try to initiate this immediately, since after the funeral is over and relatives and friends leave, the parents are in great need of support from a professional person. Their shock and grief having subsided somewhat, they are overwhelmed by guilt and self-blame. The nurse can best help them by explaining that SIDS is a disease and that it is unpredictable and unpreventable. She can explain that, even if the baby had been in the hospital or if they had checked the baby every ten minutes, its death could not have been prevented. It is much more difficult to rationalize or explain the death of a normal, healthy infant to parents than to explain the death of a baby who is abnormal or ill from a known disease. The nurse, doctor, and counselor involved in the situation must undertake a monumental task.

Professional organizations for SIDS* can provide comfort and information for parents, interaction between parents

---

*The National Foundation for Sudden Infant Death, Inc., 1501 Broadway, New York, New York 10036.

who have had similar experiences, and an opportunity for the parents to verbalize feelings and reactions. If feelings are not expressed, emotional problems may arise later on for the parents and other children.

The Toddler (Fifteen Months to Three Years)

The toddler presents a more complex problem for parents and personnel than does the infant. The toddler is refining the process of autonomy. His tasks are to develop self-reliance, adequacy, and a sense of worth [5]. The toddler is still dependent on parents and others for his existence. He reflects completely the feelings and actions of parents and personnel. If they are depressed, he is depressed; if they are upset and fearful, so is he; if the parents cling to the child and cry, he will cling to the parents and cry [4].

Separation from mother is the toddler's greatest cause for concern. If mother, his organizing person, is not with him, he becomes totally disorganized. Strange persons doing strange and painful things to him in a strange, unfamiliar place send him into uncontrolled panic. The toddler needs his mother more than anything else in the world. If the parents can handle the toddler's reactions, they should be with him at all possible times to help him face the task of dying which to him is separation.

There may be severe regressive behavior in the toddler who is ill and hospitalized. The parents should be helped to understand and accept this regressive behavior. They should not be made to feel embarrassed or to feel that there is a need to apologize. Since the toddler stage of development is decisive for a balance between love and hate, between freedom of self-expression and its renunciation, between cooperation and noncooperation, the child should be encouraged to attain self-control without loss of self-esteem. Therefore it is essential to accept regressive behavior but also to help the child return to his previous level of achievement.

The parents of the toddler should attempt to maintain as normal a relationship with him as possible. They should provide familiar toys, clothes, books, foods, and eating utensils, and play familiar games, read familiar stories, and sing the child's favorite songs. The parental methods of setting limits, disciplining, and showing love for the child should be maintained to the degree possible. If the toddler does not have familiar objects and familiar interaction with his parents, he will be totally disorganized and feel that he has been abandoned.

The Preschool Child (Three to Five Years)
The preschool child continues to develop the components of trust and autonomy but primarily now develops initiative and a sense of direction and purpose [5]. He becomes increasingly self-sufficient and assertive. He begins to make his own decisions and state his opinions. He enjoys being forceful and aggressive and takes great delight in his own energy. The preschool years are years of imagination and imitation. Play and fantasy substitute for actuality. The preschooler enjoys competition, but he has to win. This period is one of constant vacillation between strong negative and positive feelings and reactions.

In helping the preschooler with the process of growing up

to dying the parents must be extremely patient and supportive. They need much self-control, because their child sees everything only as it concerns him. The entire world revolves around him, and he cannot yet empathize with the grief of his parents. His concept of death, which may be very vague, is that of a temporary condition, a sophisticated peek-a-boo game: He is here, and then he is gone, but he always has the power to reappear when he wants to.

The preschooler may have had some exposure to experiences of death and may be able to verbalize some aspects of his experiences, feelings, and reactions and to formulate questions in relation to himself and death. In response to these expressions the parents and nurses should be as honest but as concrete as possible. They should keep in mind that the child is attempting to differentiate between real and unreal. His concept of time is day-to-day reality and that is what should be dealt with. Should the question arise, "Am I going to die?" the parents could respond honestly by saying, "Yes, sometime, but we will be here with you." They might say, "Yes, but we will take care of you." The assurance that the preschooler needs is that his parents are not angry with him and will not abandon him, even though at times in his fantasy world he may have removed or replaced his parents if he were angry or displeased with them.

The parents and nurses should provide as normal and familiar an environment as possible for the preschooler and permit him to do the tasks he is capable of doing for himself. Since he seeks independence and a sense of accomplishment, he should be permitted to do things for himself as long as possible.

The parents may be overprotective and overpermissive once they have accepted the reality that their child is going to die. The parents are angry at the loss of their child, and the child is angry at the parents for letting this happen to him. Feelings of guilt added to feelings of anger cause the parents to satisfy the demands of the child in any way they can. The child's insecurity due to his illness and his perception of his parents' hostility and frustration increase his demands [3]. If parents are not helped to work through their feelings and to set realistic limits for the child, there will be only greater frustration and pain for the child and his parents.

The anxieties of young children with terminal illnesses frequently are associated with a specific symptom, such as bleeding, more than with the overall picture of what is happening to them. It is only after some treatment directly associated with the symptom is initiated that they are able to relax. It is necessary to explain how the treatment is affecting the symptoms to enable the child to make the association and help him gain a greater sense of well-being.

Fears of intrusive procedures and of mutilation are common for preschoolers as well as for the school-age child. They have reached the stage of autonomy with some sense of identity. They are unique individuals, their bodies are very precious to them, and they are very protective of them. Young children are very much concerned about anything that may damage their body image in any way. The nurse should keep intrusive procedures at a minimum and should explain the purpose of procedures to allay the anxiety that the child might experience.

The School-Age Child (Six to Fourteen Years)

The situation of working with the school-age child with a
terminal illness, and with his parents, becomes increasingly
complex. In addition to previously mentioned developmental achievement, the school-age child has developed
self-identity and self-confidence. He has become more independent. He is able to accept new concepts, to think and
decide on his own. His parents are no longer his total world.
His friends are the inspiration and stimulation for the con-
tinuance of his developmental process.

In addition to problems of separation, pain, frustration,
anger, and insecurity, the school-age child has a degree of
understanding of his condition and his future. He is able to
share his feelings, reactions, and concerns, and his parents
must be able to deal openly, directly, and honestly with
their child's feelings and questions. They must recognize
that their child is inquisitive and eager to learn and that
evasiveness will not be helpful in their relationship with
him. The school-age child no longer likes to pretend but is
in close touch with reality. If his parents are evasive or
emotionally distraught, the child will pretend that he is all
right and does not have fears and anxieties. He will do this
to spare his parents greater pain, even though the pretense
makes his own suffering greater. Furthermore, if parents,
nurses, and doctors do not provide the information the
child is seeking, he will obtain it from other persons, television programs, or resource books.

Another area of concern to the school-age child is his
relationship with his peers. He has developed friendships
and a social consciousness. Even though he is ill and dying,

he needs to maintain his established friendships and to know that he is respected, missed, and loved. Visits and communication with his friends should be arranged.

It is important for the school-age child's sense of well-being that parents, friends, and nurses accept his behavior and reactions to death. He needs to act as he feels, even though his behavior and way of dying may not conform to standards set up by family members and society. The child needs to feel loved and accepted although he may not be able to play the role that has been assigned to him from the time of birth: that of being a "good" child.

The Adolescent (Fifteen to Eighteen Years)

The reactions and problems of the adolescent who faces a terminal illness and death are closely related to the developmental tasks he is attempting to achieve at the time. Primarily the adolescent is attempting to be independent and to establish a sense of identity [5]. He begins to become emancipated and detached from his parents so that he can function on his own to a certain extent. He is concerned with acceptance by and identification with his peers and is developing ease and ability in relating to others. Adolescents will spend endless hours in verbal examination of what they think, like, feel, and want to do in an effort to test out their identity. The adolescent is beginning to work through his sexuality in order to achieve a sense of intimacy and creativity [5]. He is also trying to accomplish the tasks of identifying a vocation, value system, and purpose in life. All the adolescent's energies are directed toward physical growth and achievement of the above tasks. His development

requires constant concentration and effort. The adolescent
period is one of storm and stress, uncertainties, mistrusts,
and ambivalence. He is constantly vacillating between childhood and adulthood. At times the stress is so great that he
needs to resort to the behavior of the previous developmental level to regain control and energy to attempt the adolescent developmental tasks again.

The adolescent who is dying and knows that he is dying
reacts in various ways. His reaction after the initial phase
of shock and disbelief is one of anger toward parents,
family, and God. He is still sufficiently dependent on
parents and family to feel that they should have protected
him and saved him from this fate. If he believes in God as
a loving, protective, all-powerful Being, he is equally angry
with Him for not caring and protecting him as He should.
The adolescent's anger is projected onto anyone who cares
for him or provides care, since he feels that everyone has
failed him. He becomes angry with himself because he feels
that his anger toward others indicates that he is still dependent on them even though he is struggling so desperately
for independence. He may feel guilty, sad, or depressed
because he cannot cope with his bitter and resentful feelings [7].

It is much more difficult for parents and nurses to provide helping care for the adolescent who is dying than for
the younger child. The young child needs and seeks warmth
and comfort. The adolescent tries to appear strong and as
if he doesn't care. The behavior that manifests his need of
love and care is such that it keeps people at a distance or
forces them away completely. His parents and friends feel

threatened, insecure, and uncomfortable in his presence. They are afraid of what he is thinking, what he might ask them about his condition and impending death, and that he might talk about illness and death in general. The approach of friends and family is usually avoidance, either of the person or of the subject of death. Consequently if the adolescent feels rejected by family and friends, he will retaliate with rejection. He tries to appear strong by a care-free attitude and denial. He may not converse at all with friends and family members and may become preoccupied and withdrawn. He may ridicule others in order to bolster his self-esteem. The adolescent has reached some realization of what life is all about. If he is dying, he is faced with the realization that he cannot have the life experiences that he had dreamed and planned [7].

The more mature and stable the adolescent is, the more effectively he is able to cope with the fact of death for himself. The older adolescent has achieved a greater degree of self-identity. He has mastered the ability to accept and value his family and friends. Interpersonal relationships are meaningful and rewarding to him, and their loss is very painful. He attempts to make the most of these relationships as long as possible. The older adolescent usually becomes closer to family and friends when he is faced with death, because he is able to permit himself to care openly and directly. If the older adolescent has established some goal in life, he may attempt to accomplish this in the limited time left to him, directing his energy toward a creative activity such as writing or an artistic endeavor. He sees this as a way that part of him will go on even after he is gone.

The role of the parents and nurse in helping the adolescent die with dignity is a very versatile one. The helping persons need to be as changeable and flexible as the adolescent. They need to recognize that the adolescent's overt behavior does not always express his real needs and fears. Parents and nurse should provide the time and atmosphere for the adolescent to come to grips with the fact that death is happening to him. He needs time for reflection on how he feels and how he is going to handle this situation. The adolescent needs information to evaluate his status intelligently and mobilize his ego strength to cope with his condition. The helping persons should recognize when the adolescent's fears and questions are such that he should be informed of the serious nature of his condition. Adolescents resent it very fiercely when information regarding their well-being is withheld from them.

The nurse needs to provide assurance to the adolescent and the parents that measures will be taken and medications given to alleviate pain. She must encourage and support the adolescent during treatments which are disagreeable or painful and explain the benefits of treatments and medications when the adolescent refuses them or sees them as useless or degrading. The nurse and parents need to recognize the importance of body image or self-concept to the adolescent and attempt to sustain this as much as possible. The needs of the dying adolescent are many and varied. The kindly help of a compassionate, patient, understanding person will do much to assist the adolescent to die with self-respect and at peace with himself.

Reactions of Parents to the Impending Death of Their Child

Parents of dying children of any age have certain problems that are universal. When faced with a fatal diagnosis for their child, parents may refuse to accept or believe it. After the initial phase of shock they may go into a phase of denial and disbelief [6]. Feeling that if they search far enough they will find a doctor who will give them a favorable, hopeful diagnosis, they take the child from doctor to doctor. The process of lengthy shopping for a positive prognosis uses up their energy and makes them incapable of coping with the reality situation. This approach also confuses and frustrates the child. The parents might be encouraged instead to seek one other doctor's opinion to reassure them and to confirm the diagnosis. Preferably this should be handled on a consultative basis through the attending physician. The nurse can suggest to the parents a consultation if their physician has not done so. The nurse should talk to the parents about their feelings and their desire to go from doctor to doctor, if that is what they are doing, and explain the negative effect of this for both child and parents. The nurse should support their doctor's competence very concretely by talking about how long he has worked in his field and the positive reactions of his colleagues and of other parents. The increased confidence of the parents in their doctor will enable them to accept the diagnosis more readily.

Another common reaction of parents is to ask the same questions over and over again in an attempt to seek new knowledge and insight. The doctor and nurse must be patient and understand that the parents need to find out everything possible about the condition that is taking their child from them. The doctor and nurse need to provide the sought-after information but must realize that the parents may not be ready to hear or understand. Therefore they will need to repeat frequently and provide and interpret information on a level comprehensible to these particular parents. During this period parents may be seeking information that will confirm their self-blame. Therefore information should be presented in a factual manner that will not increase parents' guilt feelings. If the doctor and nurse do not explain, repeat, and illustrate all aspects of the disease, the parents, just like the older child, will gain this information in other ways and will not have the explanation and interpretation necessary for understanding.

At this point in the grieving process the parents may gain support from other parents of dying children. They may feel more comfortable exchanging reactions, fears, and feelings with someone who has gone or is going through the same experience that they are. The nurse should try to introduce them to parents who have gone through the initial grieving process, have accepted the reality of their child's death, and have devised some positive means of coping with the situation. She can facilitate this type of exchange by getting the parents together, providing a time and place to talk, introducing questions and problems which she feels should be discussed, and providing information and interpretation as necessary. One way of doing this is for the nurse to sit with the parents in the waiting room and conduct informal group discussions. This method provides an opportunity for parents to become acquainted and express their feelings and for the nurse to clarify, reinforce, and interpret. After this first contact the parents usually continue to get in touch with and help each other. The nurse also can use this opportunity to familiarize parents with the organized parent groups related to various illnesses and tell them what person to contact.

Parents who are hostile, withdrawn, or uncooperative may benefit greatly from this informal discussion. The nurse can help them to feel accepted in the group by directing the discussion in such a way that they will realize that other parents have had these same reactions and have worked through them. The nurse can pick up cues during these sessions which will help her to relate to the parents on an individual basis. Parents should not be forced into expressing their feelings until they feel comfortable and accepted by the group or by the individual nurse, but the nurse can help them by letting them know she understands why they are hostile, withdrawn, or uncooperative. They need to know that this is a normal, expected reaction to the anticipated death of their child. The nurse can then help them understand that this immobilizing behavior needs to be transferred into a more positive direction for themselves and their child. They might begin by accepting their feelings and reactions and verbalizing how they feel. Assuming responsibility for care of the child also is positive behavior, and the nurse should let the parents know that she recognizes the child is primarily their responsibility. In the home the parents have complete control and responsibility, and they need to be aware that they have some control over the hospital situation. Many are unable to accept the new role of bystander, and if all decisions regarding the life and daily activities of their child are taken away from them, they feel hopeless, useless, and helpless. If allowed to make some decisions regarding the care of the child and encouraged to participate in this care, they usually become more outgoing, responsible, and cooperative.

The family and social life of the parents and siblings is completely changed when they are faced with a terminal illness and death of one of the family members. Their entire daily routine and life style are disrupted by the child's illness and impending death. The father needs to continue working in order to support the family and maintain his job. He may not be as effective in his job due to his concern for the child and other family members, and he may be constantly torn between his need to work and his desire to be with his child and family. He may become exhausted from working and then doing all the things that need to be done when he is through working. However, the job provides him with a daily routine, security, and diversion from the painful reality of his child's death.

The mother is usually the one faced with the greatest responsibility. If she is working, she may feel obliged to quit her job or take a leave of absence. She may spend all her time in the hospital or at home with the sick child. She may do this because she wants to and feels the need to be with the dying child. She also may feel that the hospital personnel expect this and she does not want to risk their disapproval. She may be so emotionally distraught that she is unable to accept and fulfill her responsibilities to her other children, feeling that she will have plenty of time for them after the sick child dies. The mother needs to be helped to see that her other children have a great need of her during this crisis period. If the children are old enough to understand what is happening, they can accept their mother's absence, if arrangements have been made for their care and security. If the children are too young to understand, and the mother needs to stay with the ill child, they should be looked after by some caring and familiar relative or friend, preferably in their own home.

In a long-term illness both parents are faced with ambivalent feelings about their social behavior. They may sit home and brood about what is happening to them. They may want to socialize or go out for recreational diversions but feel that this would not be approved of by friends and family. Very often thoughtless remarks are made, such as "I can't believe that Mr. and Mrs. So-and-So are having a good time when their child is so sick." Such comments only further isolate parents and cause them to feel guilty. They withdraw into their situation and are deprived of the physical and emotional rejuvenation they could receive from their friends and from participating in therapeutic recreational activities. On the other hand there may be some parents who, because they cannot accept the reality and pain of the situation, overreact by extreme participation in recreational and social activities. These parents need helpful understanding and assistance in accepting reality and working out a balance between being with their child and participating in family and social activities. The nurse needs to be constantly alert to the different personal and cultural responses and needs of the parents of the dying child.

The siblings of the dying child are also faced with numerous problems and reactions. They need to be told the truth of the situation according to their level of understanding. How difficult a task this is for the parents depends on the success of their relationship with their children. The parents should guard against telling the children that their brother or sister is in the hospital with a cold or flu. There have been situations in which parents have said this and months after the death of the child, when one of the siblings got the flu, he was convinced that he was going to die. Siblings usually are able to accept the reality of the situation. They cannot tolerate untruth, evasion, or being ignored.

The siblings of a child who is ill and dying usually assume or fear that the illness and death are caused by something they did, thought, or said, and they have feelings of guilt and self-blame just as the parents do. Parents need to help their children talk and work through these feelings. They can do this best by reflecting some of their own feelings and reactions. Understanding listening will be helpful in getting the children to express their feelings.

The siblings need help in adjusting to the changes in their routine. They need to understand why mother isn't always there when they need her, and they should have another caring, constant person to provide for their needs. The home situation should remain as stable as possible for their sakes. They need help in maintaining energy to continue with their school work and recreational activities. Often children are so drained by their inner conflicts and disrupted home life that they are unable to concentrate on school work. Their grades and achievement in school may suffer. They may feel guilty if they continue their play and social activities with friends. Parents, friends, and the nurse should encourage them to express their concerns but to continue their normal activities as much as possible. Arrangements should be made for siblings to visit the sick child. If the children have been friends as well as siblings, total separation from each other is the hardest thing for them to accept. The siblings need constant assurance that they are still loved by the parents in spite of the changed situation.

General Considerations and Summary

Even though death is the expected outcome of life, it is the most difficult task to accomplish with dignity and self-respect. It is more difficult for a child, since he has not matured or had opportunities for total fulfillment. The approach to death at this point in time is no longer one of secrecy and avoidance. The nurse, who sooner or later will be called upon to be the helping person for children and parents who are facing death, needs to prepare herself for this role.

The nurse should know the developmental phases that children go through and the meaning of death to them in each particular phase. She should be able to recognize behavioral reactions and evaluate these in terms of support-ive care for each individual child. She should be able to provide comfort, support, and information to parents to enable them to support and care for their child to the greatest extent possible. The nurse needs to be able to face and be comfortable with her reactions and feelings about death.

The nurse and child need time together to verbalize their feelings and reactions and to become comfortable with each other. The nurse should let the child know that he will not be left alone when he needs someone, and she should determine which persons are significant to the child and are needed by him during his hospitalization and process of dying. Arrangements should be made for these persons to be with the dying child for periods of time, even though some of these persons may be younger children in the family or friends of the dying child. Hospital rules and regulations may need to be modified if the needs of the child are considered to be priorities. When the child is in the hospital, his life style, experiences, and relationships should be kept as normal and familiar as possible.

The nurse should consult with the physician to determine what he has told the parents and child in regard to the child's condition and impending death. She will interpret, reinforce and at times expand on this information, since she has the advantage of closer and continued contact with the child.

Continuity of care is essential to the well-being of the child, especially the younger child, since he has difficulty developing trust and establishing relationships with many people. The number of nurses working with the child should be as limited as possible. Continuity and consistency of care can be promoted by frequent staff conferences, dynamic nursing care plans, and conferences with parents and family. If there is a remission of the illness and the child goes home for a period of time, continuity of care can be provided through phone calls and home visits by the nurses who care for the child in the hospital. Community health referrals may be indicated and should be encouraged. These should be in addition to visits from the hospital nurse, who primarily serves as a link to the hospital and a means of continuing a relationship which will ease the pain of the child upon readmission.

The nurse needs to develop skill and tenderness in the administration of treatments. The necessary treatments should be carried out as effectively as possible to reduce the child's pain and suffering. In concentrating on growth and development and psychological response, the nurse cannot overlook the physical care necessary to provide comfort. The older child may suggest ways of performing procedures and treatments which are more acceptable to him. At times the child or parents may be able to participate in treatments. Respect for the child as a person can be demonstrated by listening to and accepting suggestions and by letting him participate in his care as much as possible. Participation in care is one means of sustaining a degree of independence in the child.

The nurse's emotional involvement and attachment for the child she cares for should not lead to overprotectiveness and possessiveness. The nurse must constantly be aware that the parents are primarily responsible for the child and that they need to assume this responsibility in order to work through their feelings and reactions during the time of illness, at the moment of death, and after the child has died. The parents' wishes and desires regarding the care of the child should be respected, and if they are able to participate in this care, they should be encouraged and helped to do so, even though they may not perform as efficiently as the nurse. The parents should be apprised of the value and expected outcomes of treatments and medications. They should be allowed, with the help of the nurse and doctor, to determine whether certain treatments should be continued when there is little hope of improvement or alleviation of discomfort or symptoms. Parents who know the child is beyond professional help and wish to take him home to die should be helped and encouraged in this decision. They need to know what care the child should have, what problems or complications can be expected, and that the nurse or doctor will be available if they need help. When children go home during periods of remission, the parents need this same type of information and reassurance.

One method of helping the dying child and his parents that has been found to be quite effective is the team approach. This team, which has been called the "bereavement team" for want of a better name, consists of nurse, secretary, doctor, psychiatrist, chaplain, and funeral director. When a diagnosis of a terminal illness is made, the team goes into action. Each team member has his own function in this coordinated approach. The patient and family are followed by the team from the time of diagnosis, through the stages of illness and death, and during the period of readjustment as long as professional help is needed.

At present the nurse has little excuse for not being familiar with the theoretical aspects of the dying process and death.

Schools of nursing are beginning to place more emphasis on concepts of dying and death as an integral part of the curriculum. Increasingly, articles and books are being published on this topic. Many encounter groups and discussion groups deal with the subject, and research studies dealing with specific aspects of dying and death are becoming more frequent. Local and national workshops and worksessions are available for study of this problem. Death research centers have been established in various parts of the country. It is the nurse's responsibility to familiarize herself with the theoretical aspects of care of the dying patient in order to prepare herself for this experience. However, it is the experience itself that will teach the nurse how to respond and care for the dying child. Each experience needs to be reflected upon and evaluated. Caring for the dying child and his parents will never become easy, but it may become more comfortable and comforting for the child, his parents, and the nurse.

References

1. Bergman, A. B. Sudden infant death. *Nurs. Outlook* 20:775, 1972.
2. Bergman, A. B. Psychological aspects of sudden unexpected death in infants and children. *Pediatr. Clin. North Am.* 21:115, 1974.
3. Bright, F., and France, Sister M. L. The nurse and the terminally ill child. *Nurs. Outlook* 15:39, 1967.
4. Easson, W. *The Dying Child.* Springfield, Ill.: Thomas, 1970.
5. Erikson, E. H. *Childhood and Society* (2nd ed.). New York: Norton, 1963.
6. Kübler-Ross, E. *On Death and Dying.* New York: Macmillan, 1969.
7. Miya, T. The child's perception of death. *Nurs. Forum* 11:214, 1972.

Bibliography

Blake, F. G., Wright, H., and Waechter, E. *Nursing Care of Children.* Philadelphia: Lippincott, 1970.

Browning, M. H., and Lewis, E. *The Dying Patient: A Nursing Perspective.* New York: American Journal of Nursing, 1972.

Cook, S. *Children and Dying.* New York: Health Sciences Publishing, 1973.

Fredlund, D. A Nurse Looks at Children's Questions About Death. *A.N.A. Clinical Sessions, 1970.* New York: Appleton-Century-Crofts, 1971.

Goldfogel, L. Working with the parents of a dying child. *Am. J. Nurs.* 70:1674, 1970.

Guimond, J. We knew our child was dying. *Am. J. Nurs.* 74:248, 1974.

Northrup, F. C. The dying child. *Am. J. Nurs.* 74:1066, 1974.

Petrillo, M., and Sanger, S. *Emotional Care of Hospitalized Children.* Philadelphia: Lippincott, 1972.

Solnit, A., and Green, M. *Modern Perspective in Child Development.* New York: International Universities Press, 1963.

Steele, S. (Ed.), *Nursing Care of Children with Long-Term Illness.* New York: Appleton-Century-Crofts, 1971.

8. SUPPORTIVE CARE AND THE AGE OF THE DYING PATIENT

Rita E. Caughill

Numerous studies have shown that children perceive death and their own dying in ways that differ according to their age and developmental level (see Chapter 6). What we seldom consider is that adults, too, progress through developmental levels throughout their lives, from young adulthood to old age. Attitudes toward death change as much during the life cycle as attitudes toward life. As we mature, as our life tasks change through the years, our views of death modify and with them our attitude toward dying.

One of the many obstacles to effective care is overgeneralization about what the dying person's needs are. It has been pointed out [14, 16] that isolation and abandonment are the common lot of the dying, but even if one provides companionship and compassion, can one be sure of really meeting the dying patient's needs? Furthermore, can one assume that the psychological, social, and practical needs of the middle-aged are the same as, or even similar to, those of the young adult or of the aged?

When a dying patient is their own age or younger, health personnel find it particularly difficult to relate to him in more than a superficial way. General inability and reluctance to examine their own feelings about death and to determine what their own principle concerns would be if they were dying add to the problem of relating in a meaningful way to dying patients.

It is the purpose of this chapter to explore how people view death as they mature and assume different roles throughout their lives; what dying means in terms of specific problems and concerns along the way; and how nurses can be more helpful when they understand what their dying patients' underlying worries are.

A number of recent studies [1, 10, 22] have brought forth some interesting theories concerning man's attitudes toward death. Riley [22] suggests that what has long been considered modern man's denial of death is in fact only a "public silence" about it. Technological advances such as life-sustaining machinery and life-destroying nuclear weapons have forced a reexamination of man's relationship to death. The public is constantly confronted with the dangers of smoking and of driving an automobile. Such ethical issues as "the right to die with dignity," the right to withhold or withdraw treatment, are presented forthrightly on our television screens. Is it possible anymore to claim that our society denies death or refuses to consider and discuss it?

Caring for dying persons in a one-to-one relationship, however, still presents almost insurmountable problems for the caring person. For how can one discuss death as an ethical issue with someone who is directly facing his own death? How can one claim to know what thoughts and anxieties preoccupy the mind of the person dying of lung cancer, if one's awareness is limited to "cigarette smoking may be hazardous to your health"?

Obviously many variables shape people's attitudes toward death. It has been suggested [10] that attitudes toward death derive from attitudes toward life, and that the latter in turn develop out of life experiences as the individual moves through the life cycle. Kimmel further develops this idea when he states, "The historical time line that intersects with a person's lifeline is another age-related dimension that affects the individual's progression through his life cycle" [11, p. 27]. This means that age differences alone are not the only factors that contribute to the "generation gap," nor even necessarily the most important. It means that older people have experienced and been influenced by a different progression of historical events than their off-spring, and that differences in their attitudes and values exist as much because of their place in historical time as because of their chronological age. Young people growing up in the present era of space travel, computerization, nuclear power, and ecological threats have a far different set of attitudes and values from what their parents had at the same age. Today's youth cannot be directly affected by the experiences that shaped their parents' impressionable years — the Great Depression and lack of economic security, World War II and the threat to the national security — they view these as historical events without comprehending their social and psychological impact on young people of that era.

Whatever the many causes of changing attitudes, obvious differences exist at various chronological age levels. Despite the uniqueness of each individual as a distinct person, certain behaviors and developmental tasks through adulthood are universal, regular, and predictable [4, 11, 17].

Attitudes Toward Death at Different Age Levels
Early Adulthood
Early adulthood is generally agreed to begin at age twenty or twenty-one. It is a period of life beset by emotional tensions, which may often be greater than those of early adolescence. Although voting rights and legal maturity have been attained in some states at the age of eighteen, many

youths are still in school at that age and may not feel the responsibility, or take advantage of their rights, until age twenty-one or twenty-two. With graduation from college and assumption of economic responsibility, the full impact of adulthood must be absorbed and assimilated.

Havighurst [6] describes young adulthood as a lonely period of life but also the most individualistic. It is during this period that most young people marry, establish a home, start a family, and at the same time begin a lifetime job or career. The fact that they take on these important life tasks alone (that is, singly or as a couple), with a minimum of attention or assistance from others, leads to the designation of this period as lonely and egocentric.

The whole process of identity formulation which absorbs adolescents and young adults becomes a crucial issue when fatal illness intervenes. The knowledge of who one is is not yet integrated fully, or perhaps not yet even completed, so that the threat of losing one's identity and one's self is an intolerable and inconceivable assault. Few young people have had any personal experience with death and in fact may never have given any thought to the subject. (See Chapter 1.) Like the adolescent, they view death as something quite remote and unnecessary to deal with until later in life.

In a recent study I attempted to determine attitudes toward death throughout adulthood. Questionnaires were distributed to a sampling of 150 men and women. One hundred fifteen were returned completed by respondents whose ages ranged from twenty to seventy-eight years. Significant results of that study will be stated here and wherever appropriate throughout this chapter.

As might be expected, the married respondents in the twenty- to twenty-nine-year age group were most concerned about their spouses and children when they thought about their own deaths. More surprising was the fact that the younger respondents (twenty to twenty-four years old), most of them unmarried, were most concerned about leaving behind their families or those they loved and about how the loved survivors would be able to cope with their grief. Concern for themselves and any suffering they might have to undergo was deemed relatively unimportant except for the hardships it would impose on loved ones in terms of either financial or emotional burdens.

These responses reflect the emotional development of the young adult, who now identifies with a social role. He sees himself as a unique person able to relate to significant others who are themselves unique, in contrast to his childhood mentality which regarded others simply as a projection of his own needs. He is a person fully capable of loving and caring, of empathy and concern for others [11].

Another important response in the study had to do with the sense of time cut short. Particularly those in their early twenties expressed concern that "they hadn't lived life to its fullest" or that they had not accomplished "anything worthwhile" with their lives.

It is significant that fear of death itself was seldom mentioned as a major concern; fear of suffering, yes, and of separation from loved ones and from all associated with "my life as I know it." Pattison [19] claims that this is the primary problem of the active young adult — the loss of his healthy body, of his self-image as an achiever, and of his newly established family, home, and career. Regret of lack of fulfillment of life goals is especially acute in this age group that is just embarking on the path to those goals.

With the advent of the thirties, life appears much more difficult to the individual. To the woman especially, thirty is seen as a distinct turning point in her life, the advent of complete maturity, the end of her youthful spontaneity. Kimball [10] points out that the female's attitude toward life and its meaning is closely related to the process of pro-creation, which he terms "the most death-defying act" available to woman. He refers to birth as a life-resurrecting experience for the woman and feels that the present trend toward limitation of families may remove this defense against death and leave the woman in this age group more vulnerable to anxiety.

At the same time this very reproductive function con-tributes to the woman's problems when she is confronted by death at this age. Generally women with dependent chil-dren view their own deaths as abandonment of their children, and this generates overwhelming guilt feelings which are difficult to resolve. The terminal illness itself, with frequent and prolonged hospitalizations, involves abandonment even while she is still alive, and her awareness of the pain and confusion she is inflicting on her offspring contributes to her despair and grief. She knows too that she will not live to see her children grow up and reach maturity, and this is a particularly depressing realization.

For the man in his thirties, worries about money reach a peak. On his way up in the business or professional world he is absorbed with economic problems both at work and at home. His emotional investment in his family is great, but he sees himself more in the role of provider than of nurturer. The answers to my questionnaire indicated that married men in this age group were most concerned about the welfare of their families, and this was specifically stated in terms of financial security. Women, however, consistently worried about the welfare of the children from the emotional viewpoint of leaving them motherless. In both sexes the fear of pain and prolonged dying recurred frequently, as well as the enforced end of productivity. An interesting note, too, was the tendency of men to fear that they would lose control and become fearful as death approached. This was expressed by one respondent as a fear of "going out scared to death," which apparently is not consistent with the male ethic of stoicism.

Single persons in their thirties were regrettably few in our study. Those who responded expressed concern that they would be a burden to others, especially a financial burden, and concern for the emotional reactions of "survivors," usually specified as family and friends. Kimmel [11] deplores the lack of data about singles but points out that they have a wider diversity of life styles than married people, which makes them much harder to generalize about. Certainly their attitudes toward death as well as toward life would be influenced by life styles. The significant others most likely to be affected by their deaths could vary from parents and other relatives to close friends. The single person with no close ties at all is probably rare, but to such an individual the professional person becomes especially important as a confidante and a source of emotional support.

Middle Adulthood

With the forties comes a growing awareness of middle age.
Not only are the children reaching maturity and establishing
independent roles of their own, but the middle-aged parents
are becoming increasingly aware of the distance that exists
between them and their offspring, socially and emotionally.
The generation gap becomes a very real entity at this point.
At the same time that the maturing children are defining
their self-identity, their middle-aged parents are redefining
theirs. They are questioning who and what they are. With
increased freedom from the demands of their children they
discover that they have time and energy left over for themselves. Latent talents and abilities are cultivated and developed. There is a rapidly growing tendency for this age group
to return to educational pursuits, sometimes to enhance
opportunities for promotion and advancement, sometimes
to develop new careers. Self-fulfillment in new and exciting
ways is becoming a new goal in mid-life.

Optimism at this age, however, is tempered by an increased
awareness of individual mortality. Time is seen as years left
to live rather than years lived since birth [17]. Early symptoms of degenerative disease (arthritis, hypertension, angina)
may appear, and the unexpected deaths of friends and colleagues are another reminder that time is finite. Both men
and women become increasingly aware of the diminishing
efficiency of their own bodies. Women are even more concerned about their husband's health than their own, no
doubt because statistics predict an earlier death for men.

In my study the principal concern of this age group facing
death was still the welfare of children, spouse, and other

loved ones. Although their children might be grown or almost grown, the parents still were concerned that the children were not sufficiently independent to get along without them. Financial security for the survivors was an overriding problem for both women and men. More than that, however, their attitude seemed to reflect an everpresent dread of separation. This dread of separation appears to constitute a threat at all ages. While its implications change through the years, its inherent meaning remains the same.

The characteristics of the forties continue into the fifties, even more accentuated by increasing years. Awareness of the inevitability of death intensifies. The deaths of aged parents move this age group to the acute realization that they themselves are now the older generation and thus are approaching death themselves. Illness and disease are a continuing ogre threatening their peace of mind if not their own health. Thoughts turn increasingly to retirement and to reassessment of the attainment of life goals in terms of "time remaining." Thus the advent of the fifties may be a prod for many, while for others it may simply bring a readjustment of goals to a more realistic level [17].

Despite these negative aspects the fifth decade of life is a time of contentment and happiness. Persons with successful careers are aware of a sense of mastery and control, a high degree of skill and ability, and a wisdom that only experience brings. This is the time when the peak of achievement is reached. For many, personal relationships improve as well. Marital happiness increases, with the spouse seen as a valued and enjoyable companion. Friendships that may have waned through the earlier years are renewed, as people look toward future retirement and a more leisurely life in which close friends are essential to security and happiness. Children are no longer a major concern, as they are mature, and relationships with them are easier and friendlier [11]. For some, however, the reverse may be true. Marriages may weaken or degenerate completely, and parents and children both may experience dissatisfaction or even hostility in their relationship. When this occurs, the results frequently are reflected in increased health problems for this age group as well as in unhappiness and discontent.

In my study respondents in their fifties were still concerned primarily about the welfare of their families, who in some cases still included children under eighteen but in most instances meant the spouse and one or more elderly parents. But now personal death was no longer so remote, and worries about the nature of their own deaths appeared with some frequency. Forty-six percent of respondents expressed anxiety that they might have to endure a long-drawn-out painful illness. When a similar concern was expressed by younger respondents, it was usually relative to being a burden to others. For those in their fifties it was seen in terms of personal suffering and pain. For the first time, too, the fear was expressed of being kept alive, by artificial means, beyond the hope of recovery. These data seem to indicate that by the fifth decade death is viewed as a threat close enough to warrant some thoughtful consideration — or is seen as menacingly close and much more fearful than it has ever been before.

Late Adulthood

The sixties are notable principally as the years of retirement, a major event indeed to the productive adult. Kimmel [11] calls retirement "a social event without a precise social meaning." Its meaning varies with each individual, but for all it marks a transition from one social status to another. Unfortunately it usually means adjustment to a lower economic standard of living, which necessitates changes in life style to accommodate the lower income. Planning ahead, several years before retirement becomes a reality, can prevent some of the shock and relieve some of the friction the couple experiences while adapting to this major shift in roles. How well the adjustment is made not only influences how well retirement is enjoyed but has a direct bearing on the length of life itself. For some people retirement is practically equivalent to death, and we have all known or heard of the newly retired person who drops dead unexpectedly or succumbs to a rapidly progressive illness. The incidence of degenerative diseases and cancer is, of course, high in this age group, and one would therefore expect more deaths from these causes. But the subconscious tendency to equate death and retirement and therefore to expect death at retirement is probably a major factor as well. Death may occur, with or without organic cause, when it is viewed as an appropriate outcome and possibly the only solution to an otherwise unbearable or insurmountable problem [8, 23]. Kimball agrees that from retirement on, life may be more frightening than death [10]. The influence of psychological stress as a precipitating factor in the sudden death of persons with known cardiovascular disease has been well documented [3, 5, 24].

For the majority of people who survive the trauma of retirement and go on to live for many more years, one of the key factors for survival is a feeling of self-worth. Our youth-oriented culture does little to foster this, and it is a rare oldster who can maintain his own self-esteem without reaffirmation from an outside source. Some can secure feedback from the satisfactions of a job, either paid or volunteer. Others get sufficient fulfillment from peer group relationships and close family ties. No one living alone in a room or apartment without meaningful contact with others can hope to maintain feelings of self-regard for long. It is the hopelessness and helplessness that overwhelm the aging in such a situation that lead to the kind of old person that our society fears and dislikes: dependent, querulous, ego-centric, preoccupied with health, talking endlessly of the past.

Much more positive views of aging and the aged have been expressed by Kastenbaum [9], who points out that as care-givers we see only the old people *with problems* and that we tend to categorize all old people to fit this mold. Most of the research on aging has been done on institutionalized aged, who are where they are because they have physical or mental problems. How typical are they of our growing aged population? Kimmel's data concurs with Kastenbaum's, suggesting that personality patterns persist into old age and that the disgruntled oldster was discontent all his life, whereas the contented, adaptable old person probably has been a well-adjusted and happy person all along [11].

Curtin [2] points out that there are 20 million people over age sixty-five in the United States, yet the majority of Americans still do not believe that anyone beyond middle age can possibly live "productively, independently, and vigorously." Perhaps the growing numbers of retired persons (due to earlier retirements and increasing longevity) will result eventually in a more positive view of the values of leisure activities and the very real contributions to society that can be made by retired people.

People over seventy frequently express the sense of being close to the end of life in such terms as "before I die" and "one last time." Yet the elderly are neither preoccupied with death nor particularly fearful of it [18]. Perhaps, as Kimball expresses it [10], they live more in defiance of death than anything else. Most elderly people are proud of their age and even boast about it, including those who in middle years were very reluctant to disclose their age.

Illness tends to be accepted philosophically as a necessary part of growing old. Losses of one kind or another become almost a daily occurrence: loss of strength and endurance, loss of health, loss of spouse and friends — all contribute to what may be an overwhelming burden for some, but in a sense gradually lead the aged person to a realization that his own death cannot be far away.

In our study the oldest respondents ranged from seventy to seventy-eight years. The majority expressed concerns related to the unnecessary prolongation of life (or even just living too long, "feeble in mind and body") and hoped they would be allowed to die "with dignity" and without a lot of pain. Most stated they had no concern about what happened after death, but the few who expressed a strong religious belief seemed to find great comfort in it.

Lieberman and Coplan [13] found that aged persons living in a stable environment, either in a nursing home or in the community, reflected their general security in their attitudes toward death as well; they seemed to be able to face death with serenity regardless of how imminent or far away it appeared to be. In contrast, persons who had recently had to change their environment (e.g., had just entered a nursing home) had many anxieties relating to death. These investigators theorized that the death anxieties were precipitated by the crisis of having to make new adjustments and solve new problems rather than by the threat of death itself. Such a theory has great potential significance for the newly hospitalized aged as well.

It seems reasonable to conclude that the fear of death and concern about one's own ultimate end are universal and somewhat similar throughout the life cycle. Differences in attitudes toward death at specific age levels seem to be a matter of degree or of the amount of importance attached to them by the individual at that point in life. Developmental tasks change markedly during the life span, but attitudes toward death appear to modify more subtly, especially after the early years are past. Thus it is important for the caregiver to be alert and perceptive of underlying attitudes and concerns characteristic of the individual's age level.

Nursing Support
Nurses, like other people, feel helpless in the face of death because they do not understand it and do not know what to do about it. It might help them to realize that there is nothing they can do about death but there is a great deal they can do about dying. Dying is a process that is strange and mysterious, frightening, and sometimes painful. The person who realizes he is approaching death can be over-

whelmed by anxiety. If you can help him separate some parts from the whole and deal with them individually, he may gradually be able to come to grips with the total reality of his situation.

Early Adulthood

For young adults the loss of self and the abrupt end to future-oriented goals appears to be the severest threat imposed by a terminal diagnosis. The loss of self or identity encompasses the whole range of the individual's ties with significant others [19]. According to Pattison, "Human contacts affirm who we are, family contacts affirm what we have been, and the control of our bodies affirms one's own self" [19, p. 38]. He goes on to say that in order to maintain a person's sense of integrity or respect for self, his hope and courage must be promoted and sustained until death.

Closely allied to the loss of self is the loss of the future. Ramshorn [21] describes the individual approaching death as grieving the loss of fulfillment, of the opportunity to become all that he had hoped and dreamed, of possessing "time ahead."

Thus for the young adult who must relinquish his claim to the future, the present becomes the crucial time, and he should be helped to utilize it as fully as possible. He should be allowed every opportunity to be with his family and any others who are of importance to him. Rules and regulations should not be allowed to interfere with the important work of mourning he and his loved ones must accomplish. The nurse should help and encourage both patient and family to discuss the situation openly and frankly. In the study I carried out, young adults expressed concern about their loved one's ability to cope with grief following the death; if they have the opportunity to grieve with them, they can at least help in their grieving process and receive help and support in return.

The following case description illustrates some of these points:

Paul G., age thirty, had been diagnosed as leukemic two years previously. He was intelligent and articulate and talked willingly and openly of his encounter with death. He seemed, in fact, to be dedicated to the cause of improving the emotional aspects of care of people like himself, who were dying and knew it. He had no argument with his physical care, and in fact had only the highest praise for it.

"When they told me it was terminal, I just didn't know what to do at first. I knew my whole world was falling apart. I went out and walked for an hour or so, trying to pull my thoughts together. All sorts of things were going through my head: How am I going to tell my wife? What can I say to my parents? How am I going to support my family?

"Is anyone ever prepared for their own mortality? I don't believe anybody can be. No one knows, either, how they'll react until it happens. I wanted them to level with me from the start, and I think they always have — but when he told me we were down to the last drug, and if that didn't work, I might have only six months left — that was shattering.

"I've never given up hope. I don't look for a miracle, but I still have hope. I mean, I've lived this long, and as long as I'm still alive, there's hope. Maybe they'll find another drug. Who knows?

"The worst thing of all is seeing my family grieve. It's hard on them. You talk about anticipatory grief — well, I don't believe my family is grieving for me as though I were already dead. It's just hard

for them to watch me suffer, and I often think, what right do I have
to inflict so much terrible grief on them?

"They've been wonderful, though. Doctors, nurses, friends —
they can all be helpful, but in the end it's the family that really counts.

"It's important to me now to use every minute I have left. I haven't
done anything really special, just a lot of things I used to put off till
tomorrow. Now there might not be a tomorrow, and I don't put things
off. Even little things have become very important now.

"If I were to criticize one thing about the care I've received, it's
that most doctors, and nurses too, don't commit themselves emotionally to their patients. Maybe they can't afford to. But they should
at least listen carefully, not shut you up, when you're asking questions
or trying to explain your problem."

There is some question as to whether the young adult ever
reaches the stage of acceptance described by Kübler-Ross
[12], where he has worked through his feelings about dying
and is able to separate himself emotionally and wait quite
peacefully for death. Plumb and Holland [20], from a study
of cancer in late adolescence and the early twenties, feel that
at best these young people may attain "a kind of adaptation"
near the end but question whether "peaceful acceptance"
ever occurs in the young. In the case of Paul G. there is
little evidence of acceptance either. Perhaps it is too much
to expect of an age group that still has everything to live for.

If one had to choose the single word that best describes a
compassionate, supportive approach to the dying, it might
well be *communication*. Adequate, therapeutic communication. Verbal and nonverbal communication. Skillful use
of communication techniques is desirable, but even the non-
skilled can be effective, if it is honest, sincere, and from the

heart. For a helpful guide to communication techniques, see Hein [7].

Solutions to problems can rarely be supplied by the caregiver and are seldom expected by the client. What is really needed and rarely provided (or even allowed) is an opportunity to express worries to a willing listener. Many problems that trouble the dying have no solution; many questions have no answer. The dying know this, and so do the professional persons caring for them, but the latter are less willing to admit it and seem always to feel they must come up with answers. Resist the temptation, and let your dying client do most of the talking. A word or two of interest and encouragement is often all that is necessary to foster an atmosphere of trust and helpfulness.

Communication with the young adult is often most difficult for the nurse who is in the same age range. She identifies closely with the patient, feels threatened by the awareness that she too is vulnerable, and perhaps senses the patient's resentment of her good health and vitality. Yet she has the potential for the most effective interaction with that patient, since she is likely to be schooled in therapeutic communication, and it is to be hoped that she has not yet developed avoidance behavior in response to the dying. She needs and deserves support, however, and it should come from her co-workers, the head nurse, and the clinician.

Claire, twenty-four years old, had been in and out of the hospital many times in the course of a widespread metastatic carcinoma. Usually admitted to the same unit, she was no stranger to the staff. All were aware of her prognosis, including Claire, whose doctor was quite open and fairly supportive of her. The nursing staff was exceedingly kind to her but were so overwhelmed by their sympathy for her that they avoided all but the most superficial conversations, and these were usually maintained on a cheerful level.

When a new young nurse on the unit was assigned to Claire, she approached her with warmth and genuine interest. After some preliminary remarks, the nurse remained silent while she gathered equipment for Claire's bath. She then said, "You are very quiet today." Claire's eyes filled with tears as she said, "Today is my birthday." "Oh?" "I thought I would be home for my birthday, but Dr. D. hasn't said any more about letting me go." "Did he tell you at any time that you might go home this soon?" Claire admitted that he had not, but that she had set this goal for herself. She then went into a halting account of her illness, the many painful treatments, her realization that she was dying, her fear of being alone, her yearning to go home once more. The nurse, herself almost overcome with grief, held Claire's hand tightly, stroked her forehead and her hair, sometimes having to "stare hard at the chair across the room to keep from crying." Finally Claire was finished. She smiled and said quietly, "I'll get up if you'll help me to the bathroom."

Later, when her lunch tray arrived, there was a three-inch square of white-frosted cake with a single birthday candle burning in it. Some of the staff came in to wish her a happy birthday. Claire smiled warmly, "They're so good to me. They can't do enough to help me!"

She and her young nurse continued a close relationship, with Claire frequently talking of her illness, sometimes calmly, sometimes with much emotion. Her nurse found these sessions exhausting but highly rewarding in the satisfaction gained from knowing she had really helped. In the beginning, she turned frequently to the supervisor for support, but later found she needed less and less of this kind of outlet.

Claire was discharged home a week later. She died on a subsequent admission the following month.

Middle Adulthood

In the middle years an awareness of the inevitability of death develops, and with it may come anxieties about the nature of one's own death. Respondents in my study of attitudes toward death expressed concern that their deaths might be long-drawn-out and painful. They also seemed to have an aversion to the idea of being kept alive, by artificial means, beyond any reasonable expectation of recovery. These concerns were expressed in very personal terms and did not appear to be viewed simply as philosophical issues. I have heard this sentiment expressed many times by hospitalized patients who knew or suspected that they were terminally ill. Some day we may begin to listen to and believe our patients, and then perhaps we will find it easier to stop needlessly prolonging their suffering lives against their own wishes.

The story of Mrs. C. illustrates many of the feelings and fears of the middle-aged terminally ill person. Her loneliness was greatly accentuated by her physical separation from her husband and family by thousands of miles. Since her story reflects so many important psychological aspects of dying, as well as a nurse-patient relationship that is sometimes effective and sometimes fumbling, it is related here in considerable detail and in the words of the nurse who had the closest relationship with her.

Mrs. C.'s illness began in Iran, where she and her husband had lived for many years. She was treated there for intestinal parasites, without relief, and finally a laparotomy was performed and she was found to have an obstruction of the cecum from metastatic pelvic carcinoma. A cecostomy was performed, and the patient returned to the United States to a well-known cancer hospital for further evaluation and treatment. She was started on an oral chemotherapeutic agent.

Upon admission to the hospital Mrs. C. was quickly labeled a "difficult patient." She was demanding and continually made suggestions concerning her care, ranging from insistence that we take her temperature more often to recommending that the doctor call the World Health Organization to check on outbreaks of disease in Iran. She was quite apprehensive and nervous and had an occasional episode of tachycardia. She would check her own pulse and upon finding it high would criticize the staff for not watching her more closely. Although Mrs. C. was quite capable of self-care, she would insist on and expect little things, such as having her milk carton opened for her.

Hearing that Mrs. C. was difficult, I effectively avoided caring for her whenever possible. The few encounters I had with her, consisting mainly of passing her a tray or some medicines, prompted me to avoid her as much as possible. Since she was an ambulatory, self-care patient, I rationalized that I could better use my time with "sick" people, and I never felt guilty about not taking care of her.

After about a month she was discharged and went to Pennsylvania to stay with her son until she felt strong enough to travel back to Iran. But only two weeks later, she was readmitted with symptoms of intestinal obstruction. She was first treated medically with a liquid diet, then with a cantor tube and intravenous infusions. She was much weaker than before and needed more assistance with her physical care. Now that she was one of the "sick" patients, I had lost my excuse not to care for her.

From the beginning I told her I would not do things for her when she commanded me to do them without saying "please." She said that she hadn't realized she did this and apologized. She also had a habit of demanding that things be done immediately. I explained to her that she could not always expect this, and that I would do things as soon as I could. She agreed this seemed fair. (Although she evidently forgot at times!)

I tried to get in the habit of answering her call light promptly, and I stopped to see if she needed anything even when her light wasn't on.

At first I played the martyr role, taking care of Mrs. C. every day, because the other nurses thought that the sicker she was, the more demanding she was. Although I had reached a type of understanding with the patient, she was still a difficult person to get along with, and at first I only tolerated her. In a few days, though, I became very fond of her. She knew that I liked her and looked forward to my taking care of her, which I did at every opportunity.

When Mrs. C. had her bouts of tachycardia and nervousness, I sat with her and talked, and became comfortable holding her hand. She often would express fear of her treatments, and was very frightened when she found that the medical treatment of the bowel obstruction had failed and she'd have to go to surgery. I suspect that her being so far from her family and friends enhanced her fear.

The day before her surgery, Mrs. C. asked to be moved from her two-bed room to a six-bed ward. It was explained that she might need the convenience and privacy of a semiprivate room. She insisted that if there was any possibility, she wanted to go into a ward. She said she was terrified of being left with only the lady who was presently her roommate, because she too, was unable to get up and around. In order to reassure her that she would not be isolated and alone, it was arranged for her to have a private duty nurse her first postoperative night.

In surgery an ileostomy was done to relieve the obstruction. It was found that the extent of her disease was severe and that in contrast with previous reports, her cancer was rapidly spreading.

Mrs. C.'s first postoperative day was uneventful. She had been placed in a private room because her surgery was contaminated. The second morning after her operation I entered her room and said good morning. She immediately said, "I suppose you've heard the bad news." I reflected, "Bad news?" Mrs. C.: "About my surgery." Then she paused before saying, "I've got cancer everywhere." I didn't say anything, but walked over to her bed and placed my hand on hers. She said she didn't want her husband to know. I asked her why, and she said it would be time enough to tell him when she went back home, and she wished not to disturb his work. I said I thought I understood, although I wasn't sure that I did. We were both silent.

I asked if there was anything I could do before I left the room, and I told her I'd be back shortly.

Later that morning when I was bathing her she asked if I'd heard of euthanasia. I said "Yes, why?" She answered, "Well, I want to know if it's legal anywhere yet in the U.S." I told her not that I knew of. I couldn't think of another thing to say, so I asked if she wanted to talk about anything. She said no, and an uncomfortable silence ensued.

Mrs. C. was quite lethargic that day and apparently depressed. I had to use a lot of encouragement to get her to help herself at all. When I told her she had to walk, she asked why she should. I explained that it was important in her recovery from surgery. She said there was no need for her to recover from surgery. All I could say was that I expected her to recover in a few days (which I did). She did cooperate, but reluctantly.

When I got her back to bed I told her to call if she wanted any little thing, even if she wanted to talk. I told her that I might not know what to say but that I would be glad to sit and listen. She smiled and closed her eyes.

Her immediate postoperative recovery was satisfactory. At one point she became very angry and discouraged when her doctor, who had taken care of her since she was first admitted, was rotated off the unit for a month. She told me she'd be willing to do anything or pay anything in order to have him back. That was impossible, but I told her doctor of her concern and he made a special point to see her every day. She became especially bitter when a couple of weeks after surgery she developed a bad wound infection, blaming it all on her new doctor. I explained to her the possible reasons for her getting the infection, as did others, but she would not remove any blame from the doctor. She was relieved, and much more pleasant and cooperative, when her original doctor was back after a month.

Mrs. C. needed a lot of encouragement to promote self-care. She refused to walk, to bathe herself, or to attempt ileostomy care, although she had previously cared for her own cecostomy. With everything from firm kindness, to outright scolding Mrs. C. finally began to be less dependent. I think once she was convinced that she would not die immediately, and was feeling somewhat better, it did make a difference. By the time of her discharge she had reached an appropriate level of independence.

Mrs. C. had spent about four months in the hospital. She decided to go directly to Iran upon her discharge rather than spend any time resting with her children in Pennsylvania. When I asked her if she felt well enough to make such a long trip, she said she wasn't sure, but that she couldn't waste any more time away from her husband. This seemed to me to indicate a realistic acceptance of her prognosis. Then in the next breath, she said she'd look forward to seeing me during her next trip to the States two years from now.

In further discussions with the nurse involved in this case, she amplified on her own feelings, expressing her difficulty in speaking directly to a patient about his or her impending death. "I'm able to pick up a patient's cues that he wishes to talk at times," she said, "but I'm frequently unable to engage in very meaningful conversation. I want badly to be able to tell the dying patient, 'I understand,' but the truth is I don't understand, and perhaps I won't understand until I myself am dying. I hope that with increasing knowledge and experience with the dying, I will come to understand enough to be of significant help to them. For now I guess all I can do is listen."

Actually this nurse did far more than listen — although listening is one of the more important things a nurse can do. She offered herself in real and tangible ways: her physical presence, her calm acceptance of Mrs. C.'s varying moods, her encouragement and reassurance when appropriate.

Feelings of abandonment, experienced by most dying patients, were accentuated for Mrs. C. by her transfer to a private room after her expressed fear of being left "alone" with a roommate who was herself bedridden. Her separation from close family members and her alienation from most of the staff left her literally alone much of the time, and in spite of this one nurse's efforts to spend as much time with her as possible, the nurse had other sick patients to attend to and admitted that she spent less and less time with Mrs. C. as her postoperative condition improved. The final blow to Mrs. C.'s security was the transfer of her doctor through normal rotation assignments at the hospital.

One important step her nurse could have taken to improve her supportive care was to initiate a team conference. If she had shared her perceptions of Mrs. C. and her needs with the rest of the staff, it could have effected a change in attitude and improved care greatly. While many nurses give devoted and highly effective care to "problem" patients, the problem remains for the majority of the staff, and overall care does not improve at all. The time spent in staff team conferences is time well invested. It can result not only in improved patient care but in reduced staff frustration and fewer wasted efforts, a sense of achievement and satisfaction, and increased morale.

One last important point in this case is the hope that appears to be typical of all dying patients. Despite the fact that Mrs. C. at one point asked about euthanasia, seeming to indicate a desire to avoid needless suffering and prolongation of life, she nevertheless consented to restart chemotherapy following her surgery. It seems clear that she had indeed not given up hope! She also had great trust in her favorite doctor, who did allow her to hope but always within limitations. For example, on one occasion when he was changing her dressing, she begged him, "Please tell me again, Doctor. Tell me that there's a chance that my medicine will let me live." And he did. He did not say it *would* help, he said it *could* help; that there were cases of relative success with the use of chemotherapy, and he hoped that would be the case with her. She was grateful for that much.

Hope should never be denied a patient, yet it should not be offered in unrealistic terms. While life exists, there is room for hope, and the dying person can find comfort in the slimmest thread that is held out to him. Who could deny him that?

Late Adulthood

While elderly adults usually are well aware that their own deaths cannot be far away, this is not to say that they welcome or are necessarily resigned to this fact. Many have an air of serenity about them and may indeed be reflecting their true feelings. Others appear to be resigned to the inevitable, while yet another type fights death and clings to life with all the tenacity of youth.

It is a mistake to assume anything from the facade the patient presents. Elderly people (including those in their nineties) may be just as frightened at the threat of death as a young nurse is, and equally unable to cope with their anxieties. Again, communication is the key: a warm, receptive, and unhurried attitude, meeting the patient's eyes with concern, a touch, a gesture. Supportive care in itself is not necessarily helpful or comforting; it is the way in which it is administered that makes a difference.

Avoid overreacting to the elderly patient's complaints. The aged often have increased difficulty waiting for things to be done, and may become irritable and demanding. Reflect for a moment that only a brief time remains for this patient, and you may be better able to tolerate his behavior. The mere fact of having to adjust to a new and unfamiliar, often frightening, environment may precipitate marked anxiety and regressive behavior in the aged. You may never know how effectively you were able to meet your patient's needs, relieve his fears, and comfort him. But a sincere effort will be effective to some degree in alleviating the loneliness and making the dying process a little easier.

Mrs. S., seventy-five, knew she was dying and had reached some degree of acceptance even before hospitalization. One thing she seemed to fight, however, was becoming helpless. In her many cries for help I felt I could hear the entreaty, "Don't let me die alone. Help me to die with dignity and in control of myself!" In fact she did say once in a tone of fear and disbelief, "I'm helpless. What should I do?" All I could say to her was, "I'll stay with you. I'll help you all I can. I won't leave you alone." I held her close until she quieted down.

Kübler-Ross [12] emphasizes the point that when a patient indicates he wants to talk *now*, you sit down *now* and listen, as it may be the one and only opportunity to do so.

Mr. L., sixty-five, had advanced metastatic cancer and severe, intractable pain. A cordotomy and increased doses of narcotics did little to decrease his pain. He became depressed, refused to eat, and would not respond to the staff or to his wife. He continually cried to God for help, moaning, crying, and praying.

One night I went in to give him a pain shot and to try to make him comfortable. I did all I could, then sat down next to him. It was about three o'clock in the morning, and we began to talk. He talked mostly about the past and how nice things had been then and how he wished everything could be as nice now. He emphasized that the pain had been too much for him to take, and he didn't want to have to take it any longer. He was afraid. We talked for over two hours. I was glad we had the chance. I believe it helped him.

Patients often talk at length about the past, like a review of life in preparation for death. They may never mention their dying but instead savor the good times, the meaningful relations, the loving spouse, and how much it all has meant to them. Quite often they want to give the nurse advice regarding her own life, perhaps in an attempt at a kind of immortality, imparting their wisdom to another. Mrs. C., the woman from Iran, was intent on marrying off her favorite nurse, continually trying to "fix her up" with one of the doctors!

As in the case of Mr. L., men may lose their customary control of their emotions and, when unable to regain their composure, feel ashamed because of their "unmanly" behavior. It is important to accept their behavior without any hint of disapproval or scorn. It *is* all right for men to be frightened, to be emotional, and to cry when facing the unknown entity, death.

Weisman and Hackett [23] have described a phenomenon they call "predilection to death." The patient presenting this psychological syndrome is described as "one who is firmly convinced of approaching death but regards it as wholly appropriate and shows little depression and no anxiety" [23, p. 233]. He views his own death as both inevitable and desirable and may find it hard to understand why others do not see it the same way.

Most nurses are familiar with situations in which patients expressed the wish to die, appeared to give up the struggle deliberately, and finally succumbed. Less frequently patients signify the *will* to die and succeed in doing so, even though the illness that brought them to the hospital is not in itself fatal.

Mrs. G., seventy-eight, was admitted with gangrene of the left foot. A diabetic for many years, she had lost her right leg to gangrene some years before, but had been able to remain self-sufficient and had continued to live alone. She was extremely resistive to the idea of amputation of her remaining leg, although she realized there was no feasible alternative. When she was scheduled for an operation, she became almost hysterical and said she would rather die than lose that leg. The operation was postponed in the hope that she could be reconciled to some extent, but she remained adamant. Finally the surgeon told her family, two daughters and a son, that she would die if he did not amputate the leg. The decision was made to operate.

All the way to the surgical procedure Mrs. G. moaned, "I don't want to go. Don't make me go!" When she returned to the floor after the operation, she was resistive to all care, pushing people away, pulling out her I.V. needle, and so forth. She stonily refused such prophylactic measures as deep-breathing and coughing. She resisted efforts to turn her on her side for any reason, and it required the efforts of two or three staff members to move her at all, as she was a large, strong woman. Her facial expression was blank, her eyes dull, and her voice a monotone as she repeated over and over, "Let me out of here. Leave me alone. Let me out of here." The only person she would tolerate near her without protesting was her son. He was able to soothe and quiet her, but she still said no more to him than "Let me out of here."

On her second postoperative day she had her first episode of acute pulmonary edema. Although the physician had ordered "no extraordinary measures" to save her life, staff interpreted this to mean only cardiac resuscitation and proceeded with vigorous treatment of the pulmonary edema. Physiologically she responded well, but in the next twenty-four hours she suffered three more acute episodes, each time responding less and less well to treatment. In the fourth attack of pulmonary edema she died.

Physically there was no apparent reason why Mrs. G. could not have recovered well from the operation. She seemed a clear example of self-willed death, a phenomenon characterized by Milton [15] as a throwback to voodoo deaths in primitive societies. He describes two kinds of "death by witchcraft" in Australian aborigines, one in which a spell is cast on the victim, the other in which the patient wills his own death without any outside interference. The examples cited by Milton are very similar to the case of Mrs. G.: the subject simply "turns his face to the wall" and, with blank indifference to everything, waits to die.

Staff feel helpless and frustrated in a situation like this. Mrs. G.'s nurses recognized a difference in her attitude. They sympathized with her preference to die rather than to live as a helpless invalid, yet they felt strangely uneasy about it, almost as though they realized she was stronger than they were and that she would win this battle no matter what they did. People who want to live find it difficult to understand a person who is determined to die. In this case Mrs. G.'s age made it easier for the staff to be reconciled to her death, but when the same phenomenon occurs in a younger patient, it can create serious problems for staff as they grope for understanding. Weisman and Hackett [23] suggest psychiatric intervention for the patient, in an attempt to reverse psychic death. One might question, however, whether we have the right to deny such patients their right to die, particularly in the case of an aged person who views death as appropriate and desirable. It might be more helpful to provide psychiatric counseling for the staff, to assist them in gaining a better understanding of their patients' views of death as well as of their own.

Conclusion

All of us are human, and we are not exempt from fears and insecurities. But because we have chosen to devote a good portion of our lives to helping others physically, mentally, and psychologically, we should be prepared to do so from beginning to end. All of us, patients and caregivers alike, share the fear of death, but we, the caregivers, cannot afford to turn away. When we can permit another's life to touch a responsive chord in us, then we can begin to fulfill another's need, in life and in death.

References

1. Cameron, P., et al. Consciousness of death across the life span. *J. Gerontol.* 28:92, 1973.
2. Curtin, S. R. *Nobody Ever Died of Old Age.* Boston: Little, Brown, 1972.

3. Engel, G. L. Sudden and rapid death during psychological stress. *Ann. Intern. Med.* 74:771, 1971.

4. Garrison, K. C., and Jones, F. R. *The Psychology of Human Development.* Scranton, Pa.: International Textbook, 1969.

5. Greene, W. A., et al. Psychosocial aspects of sudden death. *Arch. Intern. Med.* 129:725, 1972.

6. Havighurst, R. J. *Developmental Tasks and Education.* New York: McKay, 1972.

7. Hein, E. C. *Communication in Nursing Practice.* Boston: Little, Brown, 1973.

8. Kalish, R. A. Non-medical interventions in life and death. *Soc. Sci. Med.* 4:655, 1970.

9. Kastenbaum, R. Aging as a Developmental Process. Paper presented at Conference on Aging, Buffalo, New York, June 1, 1973.

10. Kimball, C. P. Death and dying: A chronological discussion. *J. Thanatol.* 1:42, 1971.

11. Kimmel, D. C. *Adulthood and Aging.* New York: Wiley, 1974.

12. Kübler-Ross, E. *On Death and Dying.* New York: Macmillan, 1969.

13. Lieberman, M. A., and Coplan, A. S. Distance from death as a variable in the study of aging. *Dev. Psychol.* 2:71, 1970.

14. Mervyn, F. The plight of dying patients in hospitals. *Am. J. Nurs.* 71:1988, 1971.

15. Milton, G. W. Self-willed death or the bone-pointing syndrome. *Lancet* 1:1435, 1973.

16. Morison, R. S. Dying. In Morrison, P., et al. (Eds.), *Life and Death and Medicine.* San Francisco: W. H. Freeman, 1973. Chapter 4.

17. Neugarten, B. L. (Ed.). *Middle Age and Aging.* Chicago: University of Chicago Press, 1968.

18. Palmore, E. (Ed.). *Normal Aging.* Durham, N.C.: Duke University Press, 1970.

19. Pattison, E. M. The experience of dying. *Am. J. Psychother.* 21:32, 1967.

20. Plumb, M. M., and Holland, J. Cancer in Adolescents: The Symptom Is the Thing. In Schoenberg, B., et al. (Eds.), *Anticipatory Grief*. New York: Columbia University Press, 1974.
21. Ramshorn, M. T. Selected Tasks for the Dying Patient and Family Members. In Schoenberg, B., et al. (Eds.), *Anticipatory Grief*. New York: Columbia University Press, 1974.
22. Riley, J. W., Jr. What People Think About Death. In Brim, O. G., et al. (Eds.), *The Dying Patient*. New York: Russell Sage, 1970.
23. Weisman, A. D., and Hackett, T. P. Predilection to death. *Psychosom. Med.* 23:232, 1961.
24. Wolf, S. Psychosocial forces in myocardial infarction and sudden death. *Circulation* (Suppl. 4) 39–40:74, 1969.

Bibliography

Bischof, L. J. *Adult Psychology*. New York: Harper & Row, 1969.
deBeauvoir, S. *The Coming of Age*. New York: Putnam, 1972.
Jaeger, D., and Simmons, L. W. *The Aged Ill*. New York: Appleton-Century-Crofts, 1970.
Kastenbaum, R. (Ed.), *New Thoughts on Old Age*. New York: Springer, 1964.
Kastenbaum, R. (Ed.), *Contributions to the Psychobiology of Aging*. New York: Springer, 1965.
Kastenbaum, R., and Aisenberg, R. *The Psychology of Death*. New York: Springer, 1972.
Kutscher, B., et al. *Loss and Grief: Psychological Management in Medical Practice*. New York: Columbia University Press, 1970.
Pearson, L. *Death and Dying*. Cleveland: Press of Case Western Reserve University, 1969.
Schoenberg, B., et al. *Psychosocial Aspects of Terminal Care*. New York: Columbia University Press, 1972.
Schoenberg, B., et al. *Anticipatory Grief*. New York: Columbia University Press, 1974.
Weisman, A. D. *On Dying and Denying*. New York: Behavioral Publications, 1972.

Weisman, A. D., and Kastenbaum, R. *The Psychological Autopsy.* Community Mental Health Journal Monograph No. 4. New York: Behavioral Publications, 1968.

INDEX